MARKETING AND PREVENTIVE HEALTH CARE: INTERDISCIPLINARY AND INTERORGANIZATIONAL PERSPECTIVES

Edited by:

Philip D. Cooper
Memphis State University

William J. Kehoe
University of Virginia

Patrick E. Murphy
Marquette University

222 S. Riverside Plaza • Chicago, Illinois 60606 • (312) 648-0536

AMERICAN
MARKETING
ASSOCIATION

Library of Congress Cataloging in Publication Data
Main entry under title:
Marketing and preventive health care.
  1. Preventive health services—Marketing—Congresses.
2. Preventive health services—United States—Market-
ing—Congresses. I. Cooper, Philip D., 1942–
II. Kehoe, William J., 1941–   III. Murphy, Patrick
E., 1948–   IV. American Marketing Association.
RA427.M29   658.8'38'3621   77-25849
ISBN 0-87757-105-8

TABLE OF CONTENTS

FOREWORD

These proceedings chronicle a multi-disciplinary workshop on marketing and preventive health care held in Charlottesville, Virginia, near the campus of the University of Virginia in March 1977.

Interaction between the disciplines of marketing and preventive health care is still in its infancy. The workshop was a pioneering effort to explore the mutuality and the potential contributions that each can make. Participants at the workshop are agreed that the role of marketing in the delivery of health care in general and preventive health care in particular is destined to increase.

By publishing these proceedings, the American Marketing Association hopes to contribute to the development of marketing procedures, standards and principles that can be used to improve the overall health of our society.

The American Marketing Association thanks Professors Cooper, Kehoe and Murphy for their efforts in the development of the workshop, in editing the papers and for providing the camera ready copy used in publishing this volume.

Donald L. Shawver
Editor, AMA Professional Publications
University of Missouri
Columbia, Missouri

LIST OF REGISTRANTS AT THE WORKSHOP

Dale D. Achabal
Faculty of Marketing
The Ohio State University

Angelo A. Alonzo
Department of Sociology
The Ohio State University

Ronald G. Blankenbaker
Family Practice Education
Methodist Hospital
Indianapolis, Indiana

Philip C. Burger
School of Management
SUNY - Binghampton

Robert Chamberlain
Graduate School of Social Work
University of Houston

Philip D. Cooper
Department of Marketing
Memphis State University

Charles O. Crawford
Department of Rural Sociology
Penn State University

Robert Denniston
Cancer Communications NIH/NCI

Robert Eng
Babson College

John U. Farley
Graduate School of Business
Columbia University

William A. Flexner
School of Public Health
University of Minnesota

Ed Friedlander, Consultant
Office of Academic Affairs
Department of Medicine and
    Surgery
Veterans Administration

Jane F. Fullarton
Office of Health Information
    and Health Promotion

William Griggs
Bureau of Health Education
Center for Disease Control

Loren L. Hatch
National Institute for Occu-
    pational Safety and Health

Godfrey M. Hochbaum
Department of Health Education
University of North Carolina

Stanley House, Consultant
Health Activities Services

Snehendu Kar
School of Public Health
University of Michigan

William J. Kehoe
McIntire School of Commerce
University of Virginia

Mark Moriarty
College of Business Adminis-
    tration
University of Iowa

56158-77

Reed L. Morton
School of Public Health
University of Michigan

William Novelli
Porter/Novelli Associates, Inc.

Patricia Schoeni
Health Services Administration

James M. Summers
The Medical Society of Virginia

Graham Ward
National High Blood Pressure
   Program, NH & LI - NIH

Robert B. Whittemore
Baylor College of Medicine

Patrick E. Murphy
College of Business Adminis-
   tration
Marquette University

Harold F. Pyke
Kappa Systems, Inc.

George Strumpf
Division of Health Maintenance
   Organizations

M. Venkatesan
College of Business Adminis-
   tration
University of Oregon

Frank J. Weaver
Baylor College of Medicine

Lawrence Wortzel
Department of Marketing
Boston University

PREFACE

These Proceedings present an overview of the content of the First National Workshop on Preventive Health Care and Marketing, the first of the 1977 Series of Marketing Educational Workshops. The workshop, sponsored by the American Marketing Association and the Blue Cross/Blue Shield of Virginia, was held March 27-29, 1977 in Charlottesville, Virginia.

Participants in the workshop included representatives from academics, from Federal and State governments and from health delivery systems. Included were 33 participants from 18 states: 17 academics from 14 schools, 7 practitioners from 6 different organizations, and 9 individuals representing various agencies of the government from Washington, D.C. and also from Atlanta and Cincinnati.

The workshop was a rewarding experience and its success can only be attributed to the enthusiasm and devotion of each and every participant. The behind the scenes efforts of Janice Morris and Scott Hesaltine and several others provided the ground work that lead to the workshop's success.

It is hoped that our efforts in the development of these Proceedings will contribute to what promises to be a new and fast growing frontier for marketing as it joins hands with other disciplines to face the problems of our society.

Philip D. Cooper
Memphis State University

William J. Kehoe
University of Virginia

Patrick E. Murphy
Marquette University

A GUIDE TO FUTURE DEVELOPMENTS
IN PREVENTIVE HEALTH CARE AND MARKETING

William J. Kehoe, Philip D. Cooper and Patrick E. Murphy

The workshop, "Preventive Health Care and Marketing: A Workshop With Multiple Viewpoints," which these Proceedings chronicle, was the first effort nationally to bring together individuals, in a multidisciplinary setting, to review, to explore and to chart the future horizons for the emerging integration of preventive health care and marketing. The pages that follow report the activities, conclusions and recommendations of the workshop.

In preparation for the workshop, during the workshop and in its aftermath, certain thoughts or reflections occurred concerning the future development of preventive health care and marketing. These are presented here both to guide future development as well as to stimulate further conceptualization in this area.

First, it is necessary that marketing be explicated and its expanding role communicated to the health educator, prepaid health care plans such as health maintenance organizations, government officials in the health area, and other interested parties both within and without the government. It is incumbent on those in the marketing profession to undertake this task. Joining associations in the health area, attending conferences with health educators, reading and contributing to journals in the area are necessary steps to ensure that marketing's communication responsibility is operationalized.

Second, coupled to the communication responsibility, is the necessary realization that a mutual learning process is just beginning. Few marketing academicians/practitioners are cognizant of the activities, literature and end products of the health educator. Likewise, the health educator is not cognizant of marketing and its potential contribution to preventive health care. Therefore, a mutual learning process is necessary. Communication, as discussed above, is the first step in the learning process, the health and marketing areas integrated. The end product will be of a symbiotic nature and the ensuing benefits will accrue to the focal point of both the health educator and the marketer -- the health care consumer.

Third, during this communication and mutual learning process, the health educator and the marketer must realize that they both are concerned with affecting behavioral change. The

1

technology of marketing, validated on products and services in both profit and nonprofit organizations, may ideally be directed to this task. The action desired in preventive health care is a change in the health consumer's behavior, and the health educator is actually advocating or marketing behavioral change. Therefore, as both the marketer and the health educator are concerned with marketing, it is appropriate that the two fields enjoy increasing integration.

Fourth, as implied above, marketing has a decided contribution to make in the health area. However, specific areas in which a contribution can be made and the specific marketing technologies to be applied have not been identified and communicated to the health educator. Nor, has the health educator identified areas most appropriate for marketing's entry. The workshop and these Proceedings are a first step towards these ends.

Preventive Health Care and Marketing are now at the beginning of an exciting integration. The potential is explosive and defies true comprehension. In ten years, it is hoped that this integration is well under way with marketing departments operating in hospitals and health maintenance organizations, with health care marketing offices in federal health agencies, marketing courses in health education curriculums, and attention given to opportunities in the health field in marketing curriculums. There is already evidence of movement in this direction. Several hospitals have marketing officers, marketing type agencies are operating in the government (as identified in the Preface in the list of Workshop attendees), and health educators in attendance at the Workshop were receptive to Marketing. These all suggest the advent of an emerging integration of Health Care and Marketing with initial emphasis on the area of Preventive Care.

THE ENVIRONMENT FOR THE MARKETING
OF PREVENTIVE HEALTH CARE

The first segment of the workshop was designed to stimulate both formal and informal discussion. The first two papers by Godfrey M. Hochbaum and M. Venkatesan respectively, center on the place of Marketing in preventive health care. The third paper in the segment, by Robert M. Chamberlain, overviews the environment faced by Marketing on its integration with the preventive health care area.

A CRITICAL ASSESSMENT OF MARKETING'S
PLACE IN PREVENTIVE HEALTH CARE

Godfrey M. Hochbaum

My familiarity with the field of marketing has, until yesterday, been restricted to the commercial realm. Yesterday, I was exposed for the first time to a broader concept of marketing, one that comes much closer to what I believe to be useful and desirable in preventive health and much more compatible, in fact, overlapping with my concept of health education. This paper does not consider this broader concept.

I am convinced not only that a great majority of marketing experts themselves see the field of marketing more as I saw it until yesterday, but that this is the almost universal concept among all people, including health educators and other health professionals. Therefore, the thoughts and concerns to be expressed about the role of marketing in preventive health care, are likely to reflect those of many, if not most, of my colleagues in the health professions.

If this supposition is correct, you must deal with it if you want to be welcomed into and fully accepted for your potential contributions to the health field. So, in a sense, I shall hold up a mirror in which you may see yourself as you are seen by many of my colleagues. It may help you market your own profession.

Those of us who have been addressing ourselves to the task of changing people's health behavior, are keenly aware that its problems are not exactly like those found in marketing commercial products or services. There are certain differences, some of them merely a matter of emphasis or degree but some quite substantive.

There is always a risk in taking concepts and techniques that have proven effective in solving one kind of problems in one context and applying them blindly to another kind of problems in another context. One must understand clearly the differences between the two kinds of problems and the contexts in which they occur. If one understands these differences, one can select from the arsenal of concepts and techniques that have proven effective in the one setting, those that seem appropriate to the other settings, and one can modify and adapt them to the special conditions that prevail.

My personal view of the term "marketing," until now, referred to a wide spectrum of decisions and actions, all of which are aimed in the long run at increasing the sales of a given product or the utilization of a given service. Marketing includes, therefore not only decisions about how to sell, but also decisions as to at what price it is to be sold, and where and how it is to be distributed.

In respect to each of these elements of marketing, certain differences exist between the health and the commercial areas. These differences do not decrease the usefulness of marketing concepts and techniques but may demand some modification and innovative developments in the application of marketing principles to the task of changing the public's health habits and practices.

WHAT IS TO BE MARKETED

In preventive health we sell very few products--that is, concrete goods. Seatbelts in automobiles are about as typical as any. We do sell some services such as immunizations, physical check-ups, dental services, and screening programs for early detection of diseases like cervical cancer, hypertension and glaucoma. But, with the exception of immunization, none of these services are really preventive. They only serve to detect disease processes early enough to permit medical intervention when prognosis is most favorable.

When we talk about true primary prevention, the emphasis is not really on services (again excepting immunization) but on actions to be taken by consumers. And what are such actions? Abstention from tobacco; restricting oneself in respect to taking substances like alcohol and certain drugs; dietary restrictions to control body weight; blood cholosterol level and other dietary risk factors; giving up the comforts of sedentary habits in order to engage in regular physical activity, etc.

I would like to point out that these actions (that is preventive behaviors) have certain striking characteristics in

4

common: (1) They necessitate giving up things that many or most people like, (2) They are often unpleasant in themselves (at least for many people), and (3) They must last, not for a few days or even years – but a life time. Most of them mean changing an entire long-established, comfortable, and cherished living style. And, most of them are difficult to carry out for reasons to be mentioned later.

MARKETING IN THE COMMERCIAL AREA

Since the ultimate goal is to sell, the kinds and amounts of good produced for the commercial market depend usually on consumer demand. In fact, I cannot imagine that any reasonably smart manufacturers would ever deliberately produce any kinds of goods unless he has reason to believe that there exists a substantial demand for them, or that there is at least enough latent consumer interest which could be fanned into a demand. Moreover, he will package, distribute, and display the product in ways which he believes will attract the attention of potential purchasers. In other words, decisions as to what is to be marketed, are based heavily on potential and expected consumer demand.

In contrast, the health actions on which we try to "sell" the public are given to us. They are prescribed by the medical and other health professions. And these prescribed (or more often, proscribed) health practices are defined rather exactly and inflexibly. They can rarely (and even then only very little) be tailored to consumers' desires, motives, or preferences. Instead of offering our consumers things they like and want, almost all the things we offer them in the health area, especially in preventive health, are inherently unpleasant, inconvenient, humiliating, and painful; they disrupt old, accustomed living habits; and they necessitate depriving oneself of things one wants and enjoys. Moreover, there is precious little we can do to fit the product to the consumer's tastes or to package it attractively. Almost the best we can do is to make the painful a little less painful, the unpleasant a little less unpleasant, the frightening a little less frightening.

In the commercial area, it is largely the potential consumer who determines what we produce and offer, and who influences strongly the way it is packaged, distributed and sold. In the health arena, it is the health professions who determine what is produced or offered, and even where and in what form it is offered, regardless of what the consumer wants and, as often as not, against the consumer's desires and wishes. So we can see already that what we try to "market" in the area of health, especially in preventive health, is very different from most of what we try to market in the commercial area, and that the deci-

sion of what to offer the public as well as in what shape and
form it is to be offered (its "packaging") are taken out of the
actual marketing process. --You, the market experts, have nothing to say about these vital aspects of marketing.

OTHER PROBLEMS UNIQUE TO THE HEALTH AREA

As a rule, the end points of the marketing process is the
sale of a product. What the consumer does with the product
once he has purchased it, is of little concern, except in as
much as it may relate to consumer satisfaction and future purchase of the same manufacturer's products. But, the seller
does not really care very much when and how the consumer uses
the product, or, indeed, whether he uses it at all.

In the health area, the concern with use after "purchase"
is as critical as and even more critical than the concern with
the purchase itself. The person who is sold on and goes through
disease screening procedures but does not follow through with
medical treatment for a diagnosed condition, is as much of a
failure as a person who did not avail himself of the screening
program to begin with. The obese individual who has been successfully sold on going on a medically prescribed diet but is
lured back to his candy jar and apple pie after one week, is
as much of a failure as if he never had been sold on the need
to lose and control his weight. The most challenging, most difficult, most perplexing problem is not how to sell people on
health-supportive practices, not even how to get them to initi-
ate such practices. We have been fairly successful with these.
It is to persuade and help them to stick with new practices, to
keep these up conscientiously and consistently for the rest of
their lives. But which automobile salesman cares whether his
customers drive their cars at all or how they drive them...as
long as they bought them?

Let me once more illustrate by an example. We know that
the single most prevalent and most powerful motive for giving
up cigarettes is fear of disease, especially cancer. This has
tempted health professionals to use the appeal to fear of disease, and very effectively. (The skills of marketing experts
have, as a matter of fact, greatly contributed to this effectiveness.) Millions of smokers gave up smoking in response to
this appeal. But what happens afterwards to most exsmokers?
For days, weeks, months, perhaps years after throwing away the
last pack of cigarettes, the ex-smoker experiences innumerable
incidents when he suddenly craves a cigarette..A single cigarette..just one puff off a cigarette. What prompted him to quit
to begin with was the fear of cancer, a disease caused by the
accumulated consumption of thousands of cigarettes over many
years. This one single cigarette which he craves right now,

6

certainly would not contribute at all to this danger. So, the fear-motive that caused him to give up the habit at first, is rather powerless at such a moment against the strong conflicting motive to satisfy his intense and painful craving for this one cigarette.--He yields, and tomorrow this episode is repeated.. and again..and before he knows it, he is back in his old ways.

Similar processes can be observed in patients on prolonged regimens, such as long-term medication schedules, diets, and others. It is, to return once more to our automobile salesman, as if he had to worry not only about selling cars to his customers, but also about how, how often, where and when they drive them in subsequent months and years. And, the appeals, methods and techniques he would have to use to influence his customers' driving habits would obviously have to be very different from the sales techniques that led to the purchases to begin with. You can see that appeals, motivations, and methods that have proven effective for selling people on the idea of adopting the practices recommended by the health professions, are often relatively impotent in persuading people to persist in their new ways--and this is the critical issue. This is where the most critical challenge lies in preventive health.

THE PROBLEM OF PERSISTENT BEHAVIOR

Most people do prize health highly. Most anyone is eager to be and stay healthy, to lead a long life, to prevent disease and disability. We do not need to sell people on health. They are already sold on it. But, being even intensely motivated to remain healthy the rest of one's life does not necessarily mean being also motivated to do all the many things one should do to assure such lasting health. We all know, for example, that none of the millions of current smokers want to die of cancer. But this does not mean that they are also motivated to give up the one cigarette which they crave at a given moment. And the 40-year old man who knows that he could reduce his risk of heart disease (and surely wants to reduce it) by more physical activities and a more prudent diet, does not thereby necessarily want to jog or exercise daily or to give up his favorite dishes and still would want to spend his free time vigorously watching football or baseball on TV.

Of course, many people do engage in actions, even unpleasant ones, for the sake of assuring their present and future health, but very few do it systematically and conscientiously, and most people do it rarely, if at all. So, the challenge is how to persuade people to do things which most of them don't want to do but which they know that ought to do in order to get what they do want, namely that vague, illusive thing called, "health".

How often are you challenged in the <u>commercial</u> area to market a product or service which is actually counter to what people want? But, since this whole question of how to help people keep up the good works after they have started them, is itself too complex a subject to be covered here, I will proceed to still another critical difference.

THE DIFFERENCE IS IN THE PROMISE

One of the (if not <u>the</u>) most effective tools of commercial marketing is the persuasive (if not always truthful) promise of full satisfaction with a product or service. "Buy our pills, we promise, and your headache will disappear in 25 seconds;" "buy our toilet paper and it will be the softest ever;" "use Geratol and your husband will love you for ever and ever;" "let us handle your income tax return and you will save money." Note that each of these is the promise of a concrete, observable, directly experienced benefit, and that it is promised to accrue to the buyer immediately and in tangible form. The buyer is promised immediate, concrete, and assured reward for buying the goods.

But, in the health area such a promise can only be made relatively rarely because there is always a strong element of uncertainty in the outcome. We cannot, for example, promise the smoker that if he quits, he will never contract cancer of the lungs or emphyzema or heart disease; and, conversely, we cannot with any of these diseases. Only rarely can a physician promise for sure that a particular treatment, medication or surgery, will cure the patient.

Thus, people are often urged to give up long-standing comfortable, pleasurable, and deeply ingrained living habits, to sacrifice things and activities they cherish, to submit themselves voluntarily to all sorts of distasteful, unpleasant, even painful deprivations and experiences..and for what? For an uncertain and unpredictable outcome which in many cases even if it is as hoped for, may not be realized for many years. In fact, in most cases, the person will not know to the day he dies, if all these sacrifices had been worth it. Who in the commercial realm faces the task of selling people on a product like this?

OTHER STUMBLING BLOCKS

Obviously, the methods of Madison Avenue which are so predominantly based on promised consumer satisfaction, cannot be applied as universally or as simply in the health area without violating ethical principles to which the health professions adhere--or at least, to which they profess to adhere. In fact,

8

when exaggerated claims for either preventive or therapeutic power of medicine have led first to unrealistic expectations and then to disappointment on the part of consumers (something that has happened all too often), the consequences have been deep disillusionment, refusal to follow even sound medical advice, and a turning to quackery.

Yet, here we are urging people to have periodic health examinations, to see their dentists every six months, and to engage in other preventive and health maintenance practices...but very few health insurance policies cover their considerable costs. We urge people to develop healthful dietary habits, but our entire food production, distribution and marketing system is designed to prevent or at least inhibit such habits. We urge people to become physically more active but our transportation technology, city planning, architectural designs, and other factors militate effectively against physical exercise.

I could give many more examples of cases where, even when we have effectively educated the public to engage in healthful practices, the social, economic and manmade physical environments make such practices difficult or impossible. In fact, our society and its technology--even our health care system itself--seem at times to be engaged in a giant conspiracy to prevent people from carrying out the very actions we try to sell them on. This is a problem that you face rarely if ever in commercial marketing because there, as a rule, you market things for which there is (or for which you suspect to be) a substantial number of consumers both ready and able to buy.

ADVERTISING EFFECTIVENESS IN THE COMMERCIAL AND HEALTH AREA

Advertising campaigns are as a rule intended less to create (and are less effective when they _try_ to create) _new_ desires for a given type of product in heretofore disinterested consumers, than they are designed to lure already interested consumers away from similar competitive products to one's own product. Advertisements for a given brand of, say, toothpaste or cigarettes or lawnmowers, only occasionally try deliberately to sell products to people who do not yet use them. Most such advertisements are designed to stress the advantages of one's own brand over other producers' brands. In the health area, this would be tantamount to physicians or hospitals publicly claiming that _their_ medical services are less painful or more effective than those offered by other physicians or hospitals.

Except for relatively few cases, there is little evidence that the mass media do generate new demands, and that they change public attitudes, values and behavior in a purposefully intended

9

direction, even in respect to political views. Their effectiveness lies more in triggering latent audience desires, reinforcing and strengthening existing habits, and accelerating an already initiated spreading of new fads and practices.

But, even if we accept claims of effectiveness, the criteria by which such successes are evaluated, are not quite the same which we in the health area would apply. Consider a hypothetical manufacturing company whose product is bought by, say, 20 percent of its potential consumer population. If a sales campaign succeeded in increasing this volume by another five percent in one year, the company would probably be highly pleased. But, take a health program that tries to get all women at risk of cervical cancer to have yearly papsmear. If this program attracted only 20 or even 30 or 40 percent to begin with and succeeded only to add another five or ten percent to this number, the program would be regarded as a failure. Indeed, what would be proudly proclaimed as victory in the commercial arena, will often be bemoaned as defeat in the health arena. Thus, mass media sales campaigns are not quite as effective as is often claimed and believed when they are measured by standards used in the health area, and yet, even these limited gains by commercial campaigns are accomplished by enormous investments for an only slightly greater return. A large company may spend millions of dollars on sales promotion and would call the investment worthwhile if it leads to an increase in sales volume by a few percent.

In contrast, financial and other resources available in the promotion of desirable health behavior, are infinitesimal compared to those available in the commercial area. A case in point are the producers of Alka Seltzer who spent about seven times as much in 1975 to promote its use, as the entire annual budget of the federal Bureau of Health Education. (*)

CONCLUSION

By now you will understand why it was I said at the onset that the approaches, methods, and know-how that have proven so effective in commercial marketing, cannot be applied simply and blindly to the health area, especially to the areas of preventive health. Certain problems and situations have been pointed out that are peculiar to (or at least, more pronounced in) the health area than in the commercial area. They relate to what you are asked to market; to you consumers' perception of what they are urged to buy, use or do; to risks in using some of the

---

*Report at the national conference on preventive medicine, fogarty international center, NIH, November 1975, page 53.

most effective tools of traditional marketing; and to the fact that criteria of effective (or "cost-effective") marketing are more rigorous in the health area. There are other differences, too, which time limitations prevent me to discuss.

Finally, I would like to offer an observation I have often made when working with marketing experts. It has to do with the differences between health educators and these marketing experts in perception of what is to be marketed.

These marketing experts (possibly because they had been so tuned in on selling tangible things), tended to confuse two distinct concepts; promoting health behavior and promoting the use of particular agencies or facilities such as MHO's. Health administrators are likely to be much concerned with the last of these, but professionals concerned with the direct delivery of health services, with their utilization by consumers, and with people's health-related daily habits and practices, are more likely to be concerned with health behavior. Maybe, this is why marketing experts find themselves more heartily welcomed by health administrators than by, say, physicians or health educators.

In any case, the distinction is an important one for reasons which hardly need spelling out. However, while the distinction exists, the problems are of such a nature that marketing know-how, skills and methods can apply to the health area.

Many examples could be given of how these have been used and have had considerable impact on promoting desirable health practices by our public. (Unfortunately, I could give _far_ _more_ examples of how they have had very _undesirable_ impacts--but this is another matter.) In any case, there is not the slightest doubt that marketing concepts and methods do and can indeed make enormous contributions to our efforts to build sound preventive health habits and practices into the daily life of our population.

PREVENTIVE HEALTH CARE AND MARKETING:
POSITIVE ASPECTS

M. Venkatesan

There is increasing emphasis and focus on prevention of serious illnesses or accidents rather than repairing the damage
after the fact. During his campaign, Jimmy Carter advocated
that

> prevention is both cheaper and simpler than cure, but
> we have stressed the latter and have ignored to an in-
> creasing degree the former. In recent years, we have
> spent 40 cents out of every health dollar on hospita-
> lization. In effect we've made the hospital the first
> line of defense instead of the last. By contrast we've
> spent only three cents on disease prevention and con-
> trol, less than one-half a cent on health education
> and one-quarter of a cent on environmental health re-
> search. [11]

There is now increasing emphasis on prevention of every
kind -- medical, occupational, environmental and nutritional.

It is believed that significant improvements in health can
be made through changes in life style. Marketing is looked upon as one avenue to affect the life style area. Increasingly,
there is recognition that marketing can play a vital role in the
whole range of health care services offered in our society.
Recently Evanston Hospital in Evanston, Illinois created a position of "vice president marketing" and it is believed to be
the first such appointment at any hopsital. [12] Other commercial marketing practices such as special promotions and advertising to make potential consumers aware of some of their services are also being adopted by hospitals. For example, the
Sunrise Hospital at Las Vegas, in an attempt to spread the in-
coming patient-load evenly, is offering prizes ("once in a life
cruise") and Skokie Valley Community Hospital is engaged in an
advertising campaign to make the community aware of its alcoholic treatment center. [12] Hospitals have not escaped problems
similar to corporations in terms of their names, logo and the
like. An example is illustrated by problems of recognition and
comprehension created by the change of name of the University of
Iowa hospitals from "Iowa Regional Health Care Center" to "Iowa's
Tertiary Health Care Center." One of the reporters for the Des
Moines Register who interviewed a nonscientific sample of patients of the facility found that among consumers "tertiary"
had no obvious connection to medicine or health care! [1] It
may be obvious that increasing marketing intrusion in the health

care area may be timely, unavoidable and may even be necessary for the survival of the health care industry. Even the troubling experiences of the newly created HMOs attest to the lack of marketing knowledge and expertise in introducing these new concepts in the health care area. As Elwood aptly observed, "marketing has been a forbidden field for the health professional. With the exception of health insurers, marketing skills and knowhow are in short supply." [2] It is in this context that this paper attempts to present a view of how marketing can play an important role in the offering of health care services for prevention.

CONFUSIONS AND MISCONCEPTIONS

Confusions and misconceptions abound about the term "preventive health" and "marketing." The confusing state of affairs results from lack of any delineation as to what the term preventive health includes. Depending on the writer and on the occasion, it includes everything from jogging, flossing of one's teeth, innoculations for children, to early detection of cancer, heart disease and the like and the range extends to wearing safety belts and changing the life style of the individuals radically by redesigning the urban environment.

Misconceptions about marketing, its role and functions stem from the lack of awareness of the macro and micro aspects of marketing. Most of the writers point to educational campaigns and advertising efforts in such areas as family planning, mass immunizations, seat belt usage and the like to point out that marketing does not work. There seems to be little recognition or realization that the advertising or selling function (as emphasized in HMO enrollment schemes) is not marketing -- at best, they constitute a single element of marketing instruments conventionally employed by business firms.

The second type of misconception or misunderstanding stems from the view that marketing is really catering to "artificially created demands" or that while it may be necessary to market products such as shampoo, cereals and automobiles, it is not necessary to market health. One writer in the health area has asserted (in a denial of consumer choice process and sovereignty) that "the problem in the health area is not how to give people what they want, but how to change people so that they will want what we have to offer. To be more precise, physicians decide what is good for people to do and people are expected to it." [4] Some others would have governmental agencies banish certain products [9] or ban commercials on the television programs (and in print medium too) [8] in order to promote preventive health measures! Such suggestions reflect little faith in the intelligence of the masses whose welfare is presumably at the

13

heart of these suggestions! Finally, some of the misconceptions are the result of excesses and abuses by Madison Avenue and in the marketing of some products and services by some unscrupulous organizations.

There is very little awareness, understanding or appreciation of the enormous amount of activities carried out under the bailiwick of marketing management and the relevance of these commercial marketing management activities to health care areas. The important point to recognize is that marketing is a process and is performed in both profit and nonprofit making organizations. Marketing management has reached very sophisticated levels and it utilizes highly refined research tools and concepts. Thus the inescapable conclusion is that the health care area may very well benefit immensely by the use of demonstrated marketing management concepts, tools and methods.

CLASSIFICATION OF PREVENTION

WHAT IS PREVENTIVE BEHAVIOR?

It is essential to classify preventive health behavior so as to identify clearly the areas to which marketing concepts and tools can be applied. It is also essential to delineate preventive health behavior so that it does not always include the whole range of human activities relating to their life style as the focus of concern. Kasl and Cobb [5] provided a useful framework to classify various behaviors in the health area which is being widely used. Their classifications results in three categories of behaviors, viz., health behavior, illness behavior and sickrole behavior:

Health behavior is any activity undertaken by a person who believes himself to be healthy for the purpose of preventing disease or detecting disease in an asymptomatic stage.

Illness behavior is any activity undertaken by a person who feels ill, for the purpose of defining the state of his health and of discovering a suitable remedy.

Sick-role behavior is the activity undertaken by those who consider themselves ill for the purpose of getting well.

While the "health behavior" definition is most suitable for our purposes, it still needs to be redefined as it still could encompass a whole range of life style activities.

14

CLASSIFICATION OF HEALTH BEHAVIOR[1]

Some look at "self-imposed" risks such as excessive smoking and eating versus the "environmentally induced" factors. Preventive is not a discrete entity in that all of our activities have some bearing on our health. It can, therefore, be viewed as a series of overlapping sets that are not easily defined. Much of medical practice is related to "curing" which has very little to do with causes. Unfortunately, medical science has not found ways to prevent most of the diseases. There are obvious exceptions such as the usage of immunizations.

In general, one can initially recognize at least two types of prevention activities: passive prevention and active prevention. Passive prevention does not involve active participation to get prevention. Such prevention is available to the society as a whole. Examples of this type of prevention include design of highways, inspection of meat and poultry products, clorination of water, proper sewage treatment plants, airbags in automobiles, etc. Active prevention implies that the individual has some specific things to do and many of which really relate to the individual's life style. Thus, individuals must floss their teeth daily, engage in jogging or other exercise programs, buckle their seat belts, get immunizations and so on. In all of these activities individuals are fully expected to actively participate in order to gain any benefits of prevention. Even if such preventive measures are taken by individuals (such as daily exercise) there is no guarantee that diseases (e.g., coronary) are prevented for those individuals. At best, it is an attempt to change the odds or minimize the occurrence and not the elimination of the disease before it occurs nor even the question of whether one is likely to get the disease or not.

It should be observed that both the active and passive prevention measures do not, for the most part, involve the health care delivery system, the exception being immunization programs. Thus, a type of prevention which involves the entrance of individuals into the health care system and where "things" are done to them is the third type of prevention. For want of a better term, this type of prevention will be classified as "physician-generated prevention." This type of prevention is not concerned with preventing something from happening; rather the concern is for the early detection of the onset of diseases at its incipient stage with the aim of "curing" it or curbing its further progress. The importance of this form of prevention becomes clear when one realizes that even an impending heart attack can-

1. This classification was provided by Robert Wallace, M. D., Preventive Health Department, University of Iowa, and is gratefully acknowledged here.

not be predicted with any degree of accuracy even if one has just had a complete physical examination. Active prevention measures do not necessarily lead to prevention of disease but may only reduce the probability of its occurrence. Moreover, detecting symptoms of a disease early in its onset may well assure proper early treatment in most cases. This type of prevention relates to the health behavior definition in that such activity is undertaken by a person, who believes himself or herself to be healthy, for the purpose of detecting disease in an asymptomatic state. A whole host of tests and procedures administered to individuals fall in the third type of prevention viz., pap smear tests, mammaography, breast palpation, prostate examination, screening for blood pressure, urinalysis, EKG, etc.

RELEVANCE OF MARKETING TO PREVENTION

From the classification of health behavior provided, it is clear that not all categories of health behavior are amenable to introducing or implementing marketing practices. Marketing has very little to do directly with the area of passive prevention, because individual choice behavior is not involved. In the active prevention area the aim is to affect the life style of the society as a whole or at least large groups within the society. This may rightly fall under the "social change" category. Not only change in behavior is involved here, but also questions of public policy and ethical considerations that are different from those related to individual choice behavior in the market place. Strategies for social change are also viewed by many in marketing as involving "social marketing." [7] (Social marketing is defined by these authors as "the design, implementation, and control of programs calculated to influence the acceptability of social ideas and involving considerations of product planning, pricing, communication, distribution, and marketing research.) At the present time, we do not have evidence of successful implementation of social marketing concepts in changing life styles of substantial groups in societies. Evaluation of such programs must of necessity involve long periods of time. There are illustrations of successful applications of marketing techniques and practices in the usage of contraceptives in some developing countries. [3] However, these studies have involved a tangible product and marketing practices that are employed are not unlike the ones normally utilized by the profit making organizations with respect to consumer products. While "social marketing" may be applicable to some areas of active prevention, such as immunization etc. on the whole, since the active prevention area encompasses diverse and disparate activities, it may prove elusive.

It is, therefore, obvious that marketing can play a vital role in physician-generated prevention. The reasons are: (a) that the setting clearly involves a choice situation by consumers for a service; (b) the target population can be clearly identified -- that is groups that are to be at risk can be clearly identified, (c) tangible benefits of the services can be perceived by potential users of these services; and (d) the transactions take place in the market place. There are two important facilitating factors at work. They are the existence of over 150,000 well-established small and separate units of production in the health care industry and the considerable experience that has been amassed from marketing activities in the commercial sector. Finally, the problem itself is not unlike the management and marketing problems encountered by countless small business organizations, whose serious drawbacks seem to be the lack of management and marketing sophistication practiced by the larger business organizations. The need is to suitably modify managerial and marketing concepts to suit the peculiarity or problems faced by these organizations.

WHAT IS MARKETING?

Marketing should be viewed as an <u>exchange process</u>. As in any exchange, it involves two or more parties, each with something to exchange. The parties should be able to communicate what they are exchanging and to be able to deliver to consummate the exchange. Thus, marketing is defined "as the set of human activities directed at facilitating and consummating exchanges." [6] The desired exchange relationships do not come about naturally or automatically. They require skillful planning and management of the process. As such, marketing management is defined as follows:

the analysis, planning and implementation, and control of programs designed to bring about desired exchanges with target audiences for the purpose of personal or mutual gain. It relies heavily on the adaptation and coordination of product, price, promotion and place for achieving effective response. [6]

Viewed in this framework, much of what goes under the category of marketing in the health care services in general and preventive services in particular is but one element of marketing. (e.g., educational or persuasive advertising alone is used many times with very little marketing strategy involved in the efforts).

There are two aspects of marketing -- one dealing with macro aspects which relate to aggregate problems largely beyond the control of an individual organization. The impact of technology on changing existing products or changes in the produc-

17

tion processes and products resulting from technological changes
or the impact of legal environment on marketing practices in the
economy are all illustrations of the macro aspects of marketing.
These are usually treated as "uncontrollable variables" from
the view point of an individual organization. The second aspect of marketing which is concerned directly with the opera-
tions of an individual organization are the micro aspects of
marketing. Stated differently, the firm or any organization
has control only on certain marketing variables such as product,
price, communication (promotion), and place (logistics). The
planning, directing and controlling of these "controllable
variables" often called the "marketing mix", are the basic
tasks of marketing management.

MARKETING CONCEPT

The present day marketing concept views marketing as a
social process, the purpose of which is the identification of
consumer wants and the satisfaction of these wants through integrated marketing activities. [6] Such an orientation removes
the traditional view of marketing as simply moving goods from
production to consumption. Thus marketing must focus on the
needs of the buyer and not be preoccupied with seller's needs.
Some view growth of consumerism and criticism of marketing
practices as resulting from the failure of many firms to adopt
a consumer orientation in their marketing activities.

It is well to remember this marketing concept of consumer
orientation as we embark upon marketing management's relevance
to preventive health care activities. For, as the following
observations vividly illustrate, preventive health care providers seem very much the tradition of "sales orientation":

> The kinds and amounts of goods and services pro-
> duced and offered in the commercial market are
> usually adapted to consumer demand. No competent
> entrepreneur will produce or try to sell goods un-
> less he has reason to believe that there is al-
> ready a substantial demand for them. Moreover
> he will package, offer and distribute them in ways
> that he believes will attract the attention
> of people who are already interested in his type
> of product and to make the product appear as
> one that best fits existing demands for such goods.

> In contrast, the health actions on which we try
> to "sell" the public are given. They are defined
> relatively exactly and inflexibly by the health
> practices, whether preventive or therapeutic, can
> be and are only to a very limited extent tailored

to consumers' desires, motives or preferences. In fact, many and perhaps most of the actions we would like consumers to take are inherently unpleasant, inconvenient, humiliating, painful, or disruptive of cherished living habits. There is precious little we can do, to fit the product to the consumer's taste, to package it attractively, or to make it otherwise more palatable. [4]

Even the present HMOs view their marketing function as involving simply an enrollment activity -- a selling activity, which is usually planned for after all other organizational plans are completed.

MARKETING MANAGEMENT

Direction of marketing activities *is* the management of marketing in any organization. This generally involves three tasks, viz., (1) planning (strategies),(2) directing, and (3) controlling (evaluation and control). Formulating marketing strategies involve identification of target markets (often called "segments") and the development of a marketing plan, which is the selection and combination of "marketing mix variables". Identification and selection of appropriate market targets and the choice of instruments to be coordinated to reach chosen targets involve gathering and analysis of pertinent information. Marketing information systems become a vital part of marketing management. Collection of information, analyses of information and continuous monitoring of market behavior becomes an integral part of marketing management activities.

SEGMENTATION

It was stated earlier that the first task in formulating a marketing strategy is to select market targets, that is, selection of particular groups of customers or a segment of the market. Thus a market itself is nothing but a sum of these segments. In this context, target means a particular segment or segments that the organization wishes to serve. Choice of segments is based on the organization's resources, products, location and "fit" with the needs of consumers. Selection of target segments imply that the organization makes a choice from among several segments and also a choice based on those segments offering greatest return at appropriate risks. Business firms have come to segment their markets because of the realization that catering to all the segments of a market is neither prudent management policy nor profitable in the long run. So they attempt to find their "best fit" (niche) and design the marketing mix to suit their unique segments.

CONSUMER ANALYSIS - MARKETING AND HEALTH CARE

The analysis of segments necessarily involves consumers
and their needs. Therefore, consumer analysis -- their perceptions, needs and behavior -- becomes an integral first step
before any determination of segments is made. Consumer analyses involve the purchase and usage behavior of present and potential consumers, their demographic and other characteristics,
psychological variables and the like. It also involves the
analysis of consumer decision making processes with respect to
different products and services. In the health services area,
Rosenstock [10] has found that the consumers' psychological
state of readiness to take specific actions depends on the perception of consumers on their susceptibility, their perception
of how serious the health problem is and their perception of
benefits of taking such actions. Other analyses use variations
of this basic model. This is not unlike the models in consumer
behavior with respect to product purchases, where the consumers'
perceptions of the benefits to be derived from a purchase and
their perception of risk in that purchase are taken into account
in the consumer analysis stage. Consumer intentions (similar
to the readiness to act stage of Rosenstock) act as proxy for
actual purchase behavior. Just as differing segments exist for
a variety of consumer products, there are differing segments
for prevention. For example, differences in their needs for
prevention may obviously vary with age, sex, education and income. Certain age groups are more likely to be at risk with
respect to certain diseases. Suffice it to point out that identification of target segments for different services in the prevention area is possible to ascertain the needs, perceptions
and related information from consumers.

MARKETING PLANNING CONSIDERATIONS

Planning of the marketing mix and decisions regarding
which elements will be combined in what way, also constitute an
integral part of marketing strategy. The four elements -- product, price, promotion (communication) and place -- can be combined in a variety of ways and coordinated into a single effort
to reach the targets. Even if one works with only 10 variations
in each of these four elements, there would be 10,000 possible
combinations. In addition, marketing mix decisions also involve considerations of all the elements simultaneously. Also,
any program of marketing mix variables chosen and implemented
must be continuously monitored and changed so as to be adaptable
to the dynamism of the market place.

While marketing mix considerations and their formulations

20

are beyond the scope of this introductory paper, several areas of application can briefly be sketched here. For example, business firms attempt to assess the "fit" of the potential product offering by engaging in testing at various stages before a product is introduced. Concept testing procedures are employed to evaluate the accessibility of the concept to consumers and progress through prototype testing, test marketing and finally market introduction of the product. In addition, during these testing stages, information regarding the type of attributes desired by consumers, and the benefits expected to be derived by them are obtained. Such information enables the designing of the configuration of product attributes that is more likely to be successful. Consumers' perceptions of other existing products and services, their positioning in the market all help to "position" the products for the relevant segments. Considerable research time is also spent in arriving at a name, packaging and other elements related to the product. These useful techniques are applicable to arrive at a proper configuration of preventive health care services to be offered to consumers.

In the communication (promotion) area, there are choices to be made regarding allocation of resources between advertising and personal selling and between different media (media mix). Choice of media, time schedules, advertising or selling appeals, themes for advertising campaigns, etc. are all carefully chosen to get the best fit between the media and appeals chosen and the intended target. In addition, promotional schedules are determined taking into account variations in the media schedule and the need for repetition, etc. Also, the effectiveness of promotional mix and promotional efforts are constantly monitored to assure the maximum reach of targeted audience at minimum cost with maximum impact. Such lack of careful and long range planning with respect to promotion of prevention is evident if one looks at the current "educational campaigns" for immunization, drug abuse and other similar measures. Not only are these low budget promotions, but the timing, the fit between the medium and the intended audience etc. need considerable improvement. Such activities need to be coordinated with other elements of the marketing mix, which is also lacking in the present campaign for some of the prevention indicated above. For example, the immunization promotion sponsored by indemnity-type insurers exhort consumers to get immunizations for their children, but none of which are reimbursable under most of the present insurance plans (other preventive health care visits also suffer from this lack of coverage).

Pricing as an element of the marketing mix is very useful in introduction of new products or for increasing usage of presently available products etc. In the prevention area, there is no information generally available to potential consumers

21

regarding the pricing for these services. Since the "prices" are fixed by medical societies and the like and no information is available to the general public, the normal pricing policies, such as penetration pricing etc. cannot be availed by preventive health care services marketing at the present time. Such "price fixing" while not permitted in the consumer product arena is already under scrutiny by Federal Trade Commission and other agencies. In the near future, "pricing" as an element of the controllable variables will become available to the prevention area as well. Flexibility in pricing policies, combined with innovative and imaginative incentives to supplement prices will help provide integrated marketing for preventive health care services.

Finally, the logistical aspects of offering preventive health care services at locations convenient and accessible have largely been unrecognized so far. Once the configuration of preventive health care services to be offered are determined, the delivery points and methods can be developed. To make them widely accessible, policies similar to "intensive distribution" of consumer products can be formulated and such preventive services would then become available in as many locations as possible. They may well be offered at supermarkets, at the places of work, shopping centers and may even be available in "franchised" type outlets across the country. Specialized outlets ("boutiques") for specialized preventive health care services (e.g., mamography) can spring up. Increased use of telemetric devices and computized diagnostic services can result in unique new outlets, particularly in rural areas. Innovative ways to deliver the "product" (prevention) can be developed, if such decisions are coordinated with other elements of the marketing mix.

The concepts, techniques and technologies of marketing research and marketing management are already available. We also have abundant experience with their use for products and services. What is needed now is a recognition that such marketing management practices are applicable to preventive health care area and make creative modifications to adapt them to special nature of prevention. The immediate marketing problem is to make the segments at risk "users" of preventive health care services. Then the problem of making them "repeat customers" emerges.

PROBLEMS OF IMPLEMENTATION

While the relevance of marketing process to the preventive health care area may have become obvious, introducing the concepts and practices of marketing will face difficulties.

The first problem is one of attitude of health care professionals. In their view, it is demeaning to sell health. Hochbaum's observations are characteristic of others in this field: [4]

> ...it may be said that we are trying to sell people
> something they really want: health, a long life,
> and all the goodies that are presumed to be associated with health. But do we need to sell health?
> Surely, people do want to live a long productive
> life, free from disease and disability. There can
> be no doubt that all but a small minority of people
> do. People are already sold on health. The problem is something else.

Contrary to what physicians and health care professionals view as the "life giving" endeavour that they are engaged in, the typical consumer seems to consider all health care expenditures in relation to other expenditures for food, clothing and shelter. More importantly just as business firms usually reduce the expenditure for preventive health services as amenable for cuts during their budget crunch.

The second problem is one of ethical considerations. Health care professionals are genuinely concerned about what price-competition and advertising will do to the quality of health care and dignity of the profession. It is ironic that health care providers who operate and depend on the market place for their survival, have very little faith in the competitive system. If professionals will tamper with the quality because of advertising or disclosure of price and price-competition, then the problem lies with their value system and their training. However, the concerns expressed are valid and such objections can be overcome if it can perhaps be regulated as a service industry, similar to airlines as an example.

The third problem stems from the unrealistic expectations and unattainable standards that are professed for evaluating the success of any prevention program. The argument is that the criteria by which success are evaluated in the commercial area cannot be applied to the preventive health arena. Hochbaum [4] makes the following argument that many in this area make:

> Consider a hypothetical manufacturing company
> whose product is bought by, say, 20 percent of
> its potential consumer population. If a sales
> campaign succeeded in increasing this volume by
> another five percent in one year, the company
> would probably be highly pleased. But if a health

program that treid to get all women at risk of
cervical cancer to have a yearly papsmear,
attracted only 20 or even 30 or 40 percent to
begin with and succeeded only to add another
five or ten percent to this number, the program would be regarded as a failure. Indeed,
what would be proudly proclaimed as victory
in the commercial arena, will often be bemoaned as defeat in the health arena.

One needs not have to be reminded that "Rome was not built in a
day," nor can we ignore the slow increase in seeking prevention
from the most risk prone segments. Slow growth is preferable
to not attempting to reach them in the high expectation of
holding out for 100% participation (usage rate).

CONCLUSION

In concluding, it is reasonable to argue that the problems
that are apparent in the implementation stage of marketing
practices are not at all that insurmountable. After all, both
the health professional and the marketing practitioner are
interested in the same goal in the prevention area -- that is,
increase the awareness and usage of preventive health measures.
If marketing activities are likely to induce greater participation by the very segments which need prevention, then application of marketing techniques to promote physician-generated
prevention are worth a try.

REFERENCES

1. Des Moines (Iowa) Register, 4 March 1977, p. 1.

2. Ellwood, Paul M., Jr., and Michael E. Herbert, "Health Care:
   Should Industry buy it or sell it?" Harvard Business Review, July-August, 1973, pp. 99-107.

3. Farley, John and Donald E. Sexton, "A Working Behavioral
   Segmentation System for a Family Planning Marketing Program,
   (unplubished manuscript), Columbia University, 1976.

4. Hochbaum, Godfrey M., "Selling Health to the Public," in
   Consumer Behavior in the Health Marketplace. Editor: Ian
   M. Newman, Nebraska Center for Health Education, University
   of Nebraska, Lincoln, Nebraska, pp. 5-14.

5. Kasl, Stanislav V., and Cobb, Sidney, "Health Behavior,
   Illness Behavior, and Sick-role Behavior," Archives of Environmental Health, Vol. 12 (Feb. 1966), pp. 216-267.

REFERENCES (Cont.)

6. Kotler, Philip. <u>Marketing Management</u>, Second Edition, Prentice Hall, Englewood Cliffs, New Jersey, 1972.

7. Kotler, Philip and Gerald Zaltman, "Social Marketing: An Approach to Planned Social Change," <u>Journal of Marketing</u>, July 1971, pp. 3-12.

8. McKinlay, J. B. "A Case for Refocusing Upstream: The Political Economy of Illness", pp. 7-17.

9. Robertson, Leon S. "Whose Behavior in What Health Market Place" in <u>Consumer Behavior in the Health Market Place</u>. Editor: Ian M. Newman. Nebraska Center for Health Education, University of Nebraska, pp. 14-22.

10. Rosenstock, Irwin M. "Why People Use Health Services", <u>Milbank Memorial Fund Quarterly</u>, Vol. 44 (July 1966), p. 94-127.

11. <u>Wall Street Journal</u>, February 24, 1977, p. 20.

12. <u>Wall Street Journal</u>, March 24, 1977, p. 1.

OVERVIEW OF THE ENVIRONMENT

Robert M. Chamberlain

Marketing which is applied to preventive health is not clearly distinguished from health education. The apparent similarities seem to be related to the lack of open market competition in the health care industry. Although there are signs of change in other professional services, we rarely find health care services in open competition with each other. It is more likely that, like health education, health care marketing promotes a certain consumption practice without regard to a particular service source. Examples include the marketing of blood pressure checks, early cancer detection, general medical checkups, and the like. It would indeed surprise us to find Clinic X marketing its checkups as the "fastest, most painless, and cheapest in town." The lack of brand specification is similar to the industry-wide promotions of the dairy farmers which encourage milk-drinking or the restaurateurs exhorting us to take the family out to eat.

The predominance of non-brand-specific marketing in health care points up the absence of the familiar market forces. As Dr. Hochbaum noted, it is the provider, rather than the consumer, who determines the nature of health services, their cost,

accessibility, and delivery points. In addition, there is considerably more concern on the part of the health care provider
with after-purchase utilization. Patient noncompliance is a
major concern, not widely shared by other product and service
providers. These distinctions are important considerations for
the marketer entering the health field. Certain marketing
skills are more applicable than others to this sector.

CONSUMER RESEARCH

Marketing research is especially applicable in the health
care area because it serves as a consumer feedback mechanism as
well as a patient compliance monitor. In the absence of strong
marketplace forces of consumer demand and competing brands, the
health care provider has had little feedback upon which to shape
his service.

Consumer research techniques which have been instrumental
in shaping new products are clearly useful in providing knowledge of health needs and practices. These techniques can also
be used to segment the consumer population into identifiable
subgroups with special needs or social/cultural preferences.
The knowledge of consumer research could form the basis for a
more consumer-based health care system. A recent study of seven
alternative abortion services in Washington, D.C., showed that
the perceptions of patients regarding the services were clearly
different from the suppositions of the providers on several key
issues. Certainly marketing research is necessary in such situations. Not only can such research inform the provider about
the health needs, practices, and desires of consumers, but the
research can serve as a basis for consumer education programs.
The consequence of such efforts could result in a closer con-
gruence between the notions of the consumer and provider.

ISSUES INVOLVED WITH IMPLEMENTING MARKETING RESEARCH

There is clearly a stigma attached to commercial marketing
by professional medicine. Therefore, it is unlikely that marketing will succeed in the health sector unless the physicians
who dominate the delivery system are brought into the marketing
effort. The outside marketing consultant is not likely to develop the relationship with the provider which enhances implementation. Unless they are a part of the research or promotion
effort, physicians and other health professionals will not develop the interest necessary to adopt specified marketing strat-
igies. This interest in marketing can be further increased by
the concern brought on by restricted resources or clientele.
Certainly, the Red Cross is more interested in the motivations
of blood donors during times of short supply than when they have
ample donations. Financial considerations by providers and in-

26

surers have sparked consumer studies in several states. The Federal Government is now interested in comsumer utilization under various conditions of copayment.

The above examples represent the larger-scale organizations in a predominately cottage industry environment. How can marketing be effective without an organization to sponsor comsumer research and mass marketing strategies? One proposed solution is point of purchase personal selling. Since most health care is delivered in a one-to-one private encounter, ample opportunities for the physician to market preventive practices and services exist. How can the marketing discipline make this promotion more successful? One proposal is to teach some elementary marketing principles to medical students. First is learning the consumer's perceived needs, his health values, and building an approach on this knowledge. Second, the physician must learn to modify the authoritarian stance and avoid dictating to the consumer. Thirdly, the services must be made available at a convenient time and location. These examples of simple marketing techniques seem essential to marketing preventive health practices at the point of contact.

Finally, we must focus marketing skills on those environmental deterrents to good health; namely the food system, transportation, air quality, and other systems for which we have current technology to improve. Everywhere products, services, and living space are offered which may be detrimental to health. We should consider using marketing techniques to influence prepared food manufacturers and the restaurant industry to offer tasty, healthful foods. Further, we should consider marketing health interests to legislators and other influential persons in government. A broad spectrum of issues vie for their attention and every marketing skill is necessary to make preventive health a commanding subject for advocacy.

CONCLUSION

This segment focused upon the various positive and negative aspects of marketing as it might be applied to preventive health care. We concluded that the marketing discipline has much to offer health providers in developing more consumer-oriented services. Also, health providers need to be an integral part of marketing research if they are to be convinced of marketing strategies' applicability. Furthermore, unlike other sectors, health delivery organizations tend to be small-scale. Such settings offer a marketing opportunity for the physician to promote preventive services and practices. On the negative side, we noted that a large part of our environment is unhealthy and that we should develop marketing strategies to promote health concerns to key decision-makers in industry and government.

II

VIEWPOINTS ON PREVENTIVE HEALTH CARE BEHAVIOR

Viewpoints on several aspects of marketing in the health care area are presented in this section. The papers feature approaches from both the health education area (Snehendu B. Kar) and the marketing area (Philip D. Cooper) to analyzing preventive health care situations. Following these, a paper by Charles O. Crawford overviews the session.

COMMUNICATIONS AND MARKETING IN
HEALTH AND FAMILY PLANNING PROGRAMS

Snehendu B. Kar

INTRODUCTION

This paper examines and evaluates several issues central to the application of marketing and persuasive communication strategies for preventive health care programs for the public (hereafter referred to as "Public Health Programs"). The primary focus is on an evaluation of these issues in terms of the results and implications of an empirical field study. This study explores the determinants of and the means for promoting family planning methods among the fertile couples in Venezuela. The study thus has dual characteristics of a program concerned with: (1) Preventive Health Care: since it attempts to avoid harmful health, economic, and social consequences of unwanted and unplanned pregnancies, and (2) Persuasive Communication: since it deals with the means for promoting the use of modern contraceptives among those who are not users of such methods.

CENTRAL ISSUES IN COMMUNICATION AND MARKETING

In spite of apparent differences, both marketing and public health programs at one level share a common goal, that is, to change the behavior of their clients in a predetermined way.[1] However, the immediate goals of these two programs may frequently appear to be contradictory; while marketing programs are more likely to urge their clients to buy more products (such as cigarettes or alcoholic beverages), many public health programs are likely to urge their clients to reduce if not eliminate

---

1. For an excellent comparison of marketing and public health programs, see G. M. Hochbaum's paper in this volume.

28

their use of certain products. In addition, marketing efforts
are product specific while public health programs are not always.
For instance, a heart disease control program and a leading
sporting goods industry both may promote physical exercise among
their clients. The goal of marketing, in this case, is to increase the sales of exercise equipment; while the goal of a
health program would be to promote physical exercise to prevent
health problems such as obesity and cardiac attacks. While marketing success would be determined by sales volume of one manufacturer's products, a health program's success will be primarily measured in terms of the incidence of cardiac attacks. In
spite of these and other differences, both marketing and health
programs are concerned with changing consumer behavior and hence
must effectively deal with a set of issues generic to both.

The chief among these are: (1) what is the impact of level
of demand (motivation/attitude) on actions; (2) what other non-
motivational factors along with demand maximize action; (3) how
do these factors vary and thus influence the final outcome of a
program by social strata or market segments; and, (4) what are
the ethical and legal limits of programmatic interventions?

This paper deals mainly with the major findings and implications of the Venezuela study with particular reference to the
first three issues central to communication and marketing interventions. Every intervention which concerns itself with changing people's thought and actions is inescapably involved with
legal and ethical issues. However, the discussion of various
ethical and legal issues is beyond the scope of this paper, and
are available elsewhere [2,13,16]. It would suffice here to
note that decisions for marketing and public health interventions cannot be made without adequate evaluation of the legal
and ethical constraints within a specific situational context.

THE VENEZUELA STUDY DESIGN

Formally titled the "Venezuela Field Trial Project"[2] this
study is concerned with an investigation of the determinants of
fertility and contraceptive behavior, and with an evaluation of
the relative impacts of three intervention strategies designed
to promote the use of modern contraceptives among the fertile
and sexually active population. The study consists of three

2. The project was jointly sponsored by the University of
Michigan, the Office of Population and Humanitarian Affairs,
the Agency for International Development, the State Department,
the U.S. Government, and the Venezuelan Association for Family
Planning. Subsequently the project continued to receive support
from the Ministry of Social Welfare (Bienster Social) of the
government of Venezuela and the UNESCO, Paris.

phases: (1) <u>Baseline</u> <u>Survey</u>: designed to investigate the determinants of fertility and contraceptive behavior, (2) <u>Intervention</u>: designed for field trial of the three strategies (use of community leaders; satisfied users among peers; and the official workers of various human service agencies except those involved with family planning), and (3) <u>Resurvey</u>: designed to evaluate the relative effectiveness of the three intervention strategies and to compare their impacts against control areas.

The study was conducted through personal interviews of 2,446 women of reproductive ages in four geographical areas in Venezuela. A multistep probability sample design was used to select the respondents and, in terms of the major socio-economic, demographic, and fertility measures (age, education, income, fertility, and contraception, etc.), the central tendencies of the study sample are comparable to those of the Venezuelan population obtained through the national census of 1971. The field work was carried out in 1974 and the interviews consisted of 67 main items (with a total of over 200 items) dealing with six areas of fertility behavior determinants: (1) socio-economic, demographic and fertility status; (2) social-psychological measures of personal aspirations and values; (3) general fertility norms and preferences; (4) contraceptive knowledge and attitudes; (5) communication and social support; and, (6) accessibility and subjective satisfaction with family planning services. In addition the data on two dependent variables (past and current use of contraception) were obtained through multiple items in each measure. For this analysis, all the variables studied are grouped in these six clusters, and only those variables significantly related with family planning are included. The data from all respondents at risk of pregnancy (n=1,448) have been analyzed to examine the influence of various clusters of variables on family planning behavior. Family planning (dependent variables) is measured in terms of (a) <u>current</u> <u>use</u> and (b) <u>ever</u> <u>use</u> of contraceptives for family planning purpose only.

MAJOR FINDINGS AND IMPLICATIONS OF THE VENEZUELA STUDY

Level of Demand (Motivations) and Action

A major determinant of the effectiveness of marketing and communication programs is the level of <u>demand</u> or psychological readiness to buy or accept the specific products or service promoted by these programs. The level of "demand" is a central concept in marketing, and most marketing programs attempt to "match" the demands. The aim of marketing is not to "educate" or persuade the public to alter their demand structure, rather to derive profit through satisfying the existing demands. Thus, the nature and level of demand is a critical factor in shaping marketing strategies.

30

The effectiveness of a public health program, too, is determined by the level of motivation or demand among the clients to accept the use specific preventive health measures. However, frequently public health programs are based upon the premise that better health is a highly valued goal and that all people do or should desire better health. This is certainly true in the strategies adopted by numerous family planning programs, and is accurately stated by Freedman and Berelson [5] in their evaluation of family planning program records and Etzioni's [3] argument that changing human behavior through persuasion is less efficient than effective manipulation of physical and legislative evironment.

This paper examines this problem from a transactional standpoint; according to this approach the nature of the relationship between the personal and situational factors is what determines the health action. The results of the Venezuela study (Tables 1 and 2) show that while favorable attitude is significantly related with contraception, it alone is not a sufficient condition for the maximum level of acceptance observed. The results support the hypothesis that family planning is determined by several factors rather than by one dominant determinant category (Table 1). Of all the independent variables, perceived "social support" and "specific family planning attitudes" are the best predictors of the variance of family planning behavior, followed by "subjective accessibility" of family planning services.

Table 2 presents findings of considerable significance to such a strategy analysis. The results show that when all the three major indications (attitude, social support, and accessibility) are highly favorable, the level of use varies remarkably. When personal intention (measure of attitude number) alone is most favorable, 48.1 percent of the respondents practiced family planning; with accessibility of services alone most favorable, the practice level is 47.9 percent; and with social support for contraception alone most favorable, the use level is 67.8 percent. Thus, if the success of a program requires that an overwhelming majority of the total client population (70 to 90 percent) must accept contraception, then an intervention strategy must emphasize all three points of intervention simultaneously. Emphasis on promoting only the demand (attitude/motivation), or supply (accessibility), or social support would be ineffective.

Also, the socio-economic and demographic variables rank rather low as the correlates of family planning. This is likely due to the fact that the sample was designed to represent the highly homogeneous population of Venezuela. Had a population been greatly heterogeneous, then the impact of socio-economic and demographic variables on family planning probably would have been more pronounced.

The results suggest that within a relatively homogeneous population attitudinal and cognitive determinants may have greater influence than socio-economic variables on family planning behavior.

TABLE 1

MULTIPLE CORRELATION COEFFICIENTS OF INDEPENDENT

VARIABLES WITH FAMILY PLANNING

Multiple Correlation Coefficients of Independent Variables (INDICES)	Ever Use	Current Use
Social Support (SOC. SUPP.)	.493	.452
Family Planning Attitude (FP. ATT.)	.494	.428
Subjective Accessibility (SUB. ACC.)	.382	.365
Socio-Economic Status (SES)	.243	.206
Personal Aspirations (P. ASP.)	.186	.121
Ideal Family Size (I. FAM. SZ.)	-.060*	-.053*
All Independent Variables Studied	.603	.543

*$p > .05$

Social Support and Locus of Decisions

Individuals have very little to fear if the actions they must take to satisfy their motivations are not deviations from the established norm or the model behavior of the society at large. On the other hand, if the goal of a program is to promote a behavior which is unconventional, controversial, or is at variance from the established social norm, then the level of social support from peers and reference groups could be a major determinant in the practice of such a behavior. Thus a marketing program which promotes a particular brand of toothbrush in a society which values toothbrushing, is dealing with an entirely different situation than the challenge faced by a family planning program in a traditional or a Catholic society. In the absence of actual or perceived social suport the fear of social isolation or reprimand may be a major deterrent for individuals to act according to their personal motivations.

The second element within the broader context of social support (or influence) is the question of the locus of health decisions. Most social research in public health in the tradition of western concepts of modern man uses a molecular approach; the implicit assumption is that individuals act on their own and according to their free will. This may be true in societies in which individualism is highly valued and the actions by individuals conform to the socially approved pattern of behavior. The assumption need not be valid in those societies in which the major decisions are largely influenced by the traditional institution of family structure or the collective kinship or social units. It would not be very convincing to argue that in a traditional society such as rural India, where marriages are still arranged and determined by the decisions of elder members of the extended family, a young bride would be free to decide how many children she wants, when she wants them, and what method she wants to use to regulate her fertility. In less dramatic and more prevalent situations such as in most of the urbanized societies, this question could be formulated in a much broader fashion that is: "What is the locus of health decisions? Whose attitudes have greater influences on family planning? Wives? Husbands? Both?"

The results in Table 2 show that in addition to personal attitudes, social support is a very significant determinant of contraception, and that the combined influence of the three ranking factors is much higher than the influence of any of these. These findings have significant policy implications. First: when any one of the three conditions is highly favorable, the contraception rates vary between 48 to 64 percent (column one). Thus if a contraception rate within this range is acceptable for a "successful" program, then the choice of any one of the three intervention alternatives (i.e., promoting attitudes or demands, accessibility of services, and social support for contraception), would be appropriate. Second: when one of the three conditions is highly favorable then by concentrating efforts on a second area, the acceptance rate can be improved dramatically. For instance, when accessibility is high, by adding high social support, the acceptance rate nearly doubles (from 47.9 to 84.3 percent, Table 2). In such a situation, efforts to further augment the accessibility would be less productive than an intervention designed to strengthen a second area of determinants (either social support, or attitudes/demands). The general implication of these findings is that when one of the basic three conditions is highly favorable, a program would gain most by concentrating on strengthening the second and third component of determinants rather than by investing its limited resources in an area which is already favorable. This requires a careful assessment of the extent to which each of the three conditions is amenable to change through program efforts, the cost involved, and the relative expected benefits of each.

Let us consider the situation, in which the attitude for contraception is highly favorable, but in order to be successful, our program must achieve an acceptance rate considerably in excess of about 48 percent (Table 2: attitude is high but other conditions are low). The data also suggest that, if the program can add a second favorable condition either by creating a high social support or high accessibility, the acceptance rate would increase to 73 and 77 percents. If this increased level is acceptable as "successful" program achievement, then the issue an intervention strategist must resolve is: which of the two alternative points of interventions (social support and accessibility) is more amenable to change through programmatic efforts. One could conceivably encounter situations in which further improvement for accessibility would require a major improvement in the overall health care delivery system (the system through which, in most cases, the family planning services are made available to clients) and that such drastic improvement of the health care infrastructure and services is neither feasible nor within the direct control of a family planning program. (Incidentally, in most of the industrially less developed countries this is the norm rather than the exception.) In such situations, what could a family planning program planner do? Attempts to alter the overall health care system which is not manipulable by a family planning program, can only cause frustrations and failures. In such a situation, it would be desirable to concentrate efforts on improving the other feasible and manipulable determinants.

TABLE 2

PERCENT USERS OF FAMILY PLANNING

BY VARIOUS COMBINATIONS OF

SOCIAL SUPPORT (SS), ACCESSIBILITY (ACC), AND ATTITUDES (ATT)*

Combinations of Determinants	Attitude 1: To Use FP	Attitude 2: Will Recommend FP To Friends
Three Conditions High:		
Attitude, Social Support, Accessibility	90.0	89.8
Two Conditions High:		
Attitude & Social Support	73.1	73.4
Attitude & Accessibility	77.1	72.0
Social Support & Accessibility	84.3	83.6
One Condition High:		
Social Support Only	67.8	59.3
Attitude Only	48.1	30.4
Accessibility Only	47.9	46.8
All Conditions Unfavorable or Low	28.2	18.7

*Two measures of attitudes have been used for the analysis.
    Attitude 1: Personal willingness and intention to use the
                available contraception.
    Attitude 2: Willingness to recommend the use of their meth-
                od to friends and peers like themselves.

Another issue relevant to the decisions for alternatives for intervention is, since some people will use family planning even without a program, how much of the total contraceptive behavior can be attributed to the program? Our data (Table 2) show that even when all three conditions are low, the acceptance rate in one case is about 19 percent. This raises two questions: first, in a given population what is the proportion of couples who will use family planning regardless of a program, and second, if a program fails to achieve a rate much higher than this level, then do we need a program? If after considerable time and effort, a program achieves a 25 percent acceptance rate of which about 19 percent would have occured anyway, how effective is the program? Should a program, instead of spreading its resources thinly over the entire population, carefully choose certain segments of the population in which, by a marginal increase of effort, the acceptance rate would increase much beyond this 19 or 25 percent levels? The result suggests that, the knowledge of the level of expected behavior among the client without or prior to an intervantion, has a central place in the determination of whether and where intervention efforts should concentrate.

Specificity, Salience, and Situation

An intervention may succeed in promoting a general goal or message, and yet fail to influence specific actions. Many national family planning programs have invested enormous resources in promoting the notion that a small family is desirable; slogans such as "A small family is a happy family," or "Your future is in your hands; plan your family," were very common and reached most couples through the mass media. Yet acceptance of family planning remains at a level much lower than the people's awareness and generally favorable attitude towards the concept of fertility control. Similar experience abounds in the area of health programs; while most people approve and desire "good health", such generalized goals often fail to influence specific health actions. These are (1) generality (or specificity) of the goal of communication, (2) conflict between two salient goals, and (3) situational context of the action.

The Venezuela data indicate that as compared to specific attitudes and action intentions, generalized attitude toward family planning and ideal family size are much poorer predictors of contraception. In this study the users and non-users do not vary in their concept of ideal family size; this is likely because this measure may represent an ideal or abstract norm, while actions are concurrently influenced by many other forces in a specific situation (Table 3). The respondent's attitude toward family planning in general is a somewhat better predictor than their ideal family size; however their personal attitude

36

TABLE 3

SELECTED CORRELATES OF FAMILY PLANNING USE

Selected Measures	Zero Order Correlation Coefficients	
	Current Use	Ever Use
Ideal Family Size	-.028 ns	-.017 ns
Approval of FP in general	.033 ns	.043
Personal attitude towards FP	.313	.357
Recommend FP to friends	.292	.341
Approval of FP by spouse	.296	.341
Approval of FP by friends	.255	.268
Discussion with spouse	.336	.415
Discussion with friends	.119	.165
Distance from clinic	-.055	-.016 ns
Convenience of FP supplies	.170	.208

ns = not significant at .05 level

and intentions to use family planning is by far the best of these three predictors. A second measure of a specific attitude (whether they will recommend the use of available family planning methods) also is a better predictor than ideal family size and generalized approval of the concept of family planning.

The results imply that, due to such gap between the acceptance and approval of a general goal and specific actions, the success of a program, in the final analysis, would be the level of specificity of the goals and actions this program promotes. The now famous family planning "KAP-Gap" (the gaps between Knowledge, Attitudes, and Practices) observed in numerous countries underscores the importance of the specificity of goals and attitudes on the client's behavior [5].

In addition to specificity of a goal, its importance to the person (priority) and its relationship with other important goals (congruity or conflict), may have independent effects on actions. The importance of salience of a goal (defined here in terms of importance and congruity of a goal in relationship between the respondents desire for additional children and their contraceptive behavior. Two findings of the Venezuela study are particularly relevant to the importance of salience on action: (1) of those who want more children, 62 percent are current users and 38 percent are non-users of family planning, and (2) of those who do not want more children, 56 percent are currently users and 44 percent are non-users of family planning (x^2=38.1, p<.001). Further examination reveals that most of those respondents who want to have additional children and still are current users of family planning are temporarily postponing pregnancy since childbearing may seriously interfere with their career and other goals. On the other hand, most of those who do not want more children and yet do not use contraception, do so because either they believe that they are sterile (belief in personal susceptibility) or one of the two spouses object to the method available, or are temporarily sexually inactive due to illness or absence of a spouse. Then there is a sizable proportion of cases in each of these two subgroups, whose own desire for additional children conflict with their spouses desire for additional children.

Data presented earlier (Table 2) showed that when personal attitude alone is favorable, the acceptance rate is much lower than when in addition to personal attitudes, social support is also highly favorable. Table 3 shows significant relationships between family planning behavior and approval and the level of discussions of family planning among spouses and friends. These results considered together suggest that, in addition to personal desire for an action (attitude toward family planning), the extent to which the action conforms or conflicts with other

38

goals, and the degree of social approval or influence also exert independent influences on contraceptions.

Situational Influence

In addition to personal motivation (often specifically defined as attitude towards specific action) and social support, several situational factors may significantly influence whether or not persons would act in accordance to their wants and preferences. Even when a person desires a goal, certain situations may obviate the need for or prevent an action. For instance, there are many women who do not want additional children and yet do not practice contraception due to situational factors such as perceived or actual sterility, or temporary abstinence (due to illness or separation from spouse), or lack of accessibility of contraceptive facilities.

Recent exploratory studies among college women in a liberal campus of a major American university showed that a majority of the single college women had at least once exposed themselves to the risk of pregnancy by not using contraceptives [15, 18]. In addition to cognitive factors (such as lack of knowledge or the belief that they are not susceptible to pregnancy) situational factors played a major role in these cases of unprotected pregnancy risk. These studies showed that most women with steady partners do use contraception. On the other hand, a most vulnerable woman would be one who has just arrived at a new campus, is lonesome in the absence of any intimate relationship, is not anticipating sexual intercourse, but suddenly finds herself in a situation which rapidly leads to sexual intercourse. Often there is no time or opportunity to obtain non-prescription contraceptives let alone those methods which require an appointment with a physician and a waiting time averaging up to 8 to 10 weeks. In most of these cases situational factors play a dominant role in determining whether or not these women would use contraception regardless of their personal desire to avoid pregnancies.

Additional data on the relationship between convenience and distance of the family planning clinic (Table 3) provides further justification of the need for consideration of the situational factors for effective intervention strategy. Hochbaum's [9] original study of the factors which determine public participation in tuberculosis screening programs, and subsequent studies [7, 12, 17] clearly demonstrate the importance of the situational factors on preventive health actions.

Intervention Impact by Population Segmentation

While an examination of a population at large (aggregate

data analysis) may suggest certain variables as major determinants of a behavior, these factors need not have equal influence on this behavior in different strata or segments of the population. Thus, while social support, family planning attitudes, and accessibility emerge as the three major determinants for our entire study population, it is necessary to examine the extent to which these factors influence family planning behavior in various segments of the population. If the impacts of these factors (on family planning) vary considerably by various population segments, it would mean that one common strategy would not be equally effective with peoples in different population segments, therefore such a strategy would not likely produce the maximum overall outcome. It is essential in such cases to design a strategy which appropriately emphasized different aspects in various population segments. The field of marketing is particularly sensitive to the variation of "demand" by various market segmentation and has accumulated considerable experience in effectively dealing with the segmentation strategy. This experience would be particularly helpful in designing effective intervention strategies for public health programs.

Analysis[3] of data by population segments confirms that the impacts of social support, personal attitudes, and accessibility on family planning vary by educational status and parity (number of living children) of the respondents. Since amongst all socio-economic and demographic variables measured, education and parity had the strongest influence on family planning, these two variables were used to stratify the respondents. Figure 1 presents the percent users of family planning by various combinations of the three determinants (social support, accessibility, and attitudes) in population segments by education and parity.

Several significant findings with policy implications can be noted. First, while social support, family planning attitudes, and accessibility are the three most significant determinants of family planning at the aggregate level, these three factors do not affect the contraceptive behavior of the respondents with high education and low parity. This implies that a program which aims to change any or all of these three conditions will not likely have any significant impact on contracep-

---

3. For this analysis, the educational status was dichotomized into high and low categories; parity was trichotomized into high (with six or more children), medium (two to five children), and low (one or less children). This produced six segments of population by various combinations of education-parity status. However, the respondents in the high parity-high education segment were very few and were combined with those with high education-medium parity.

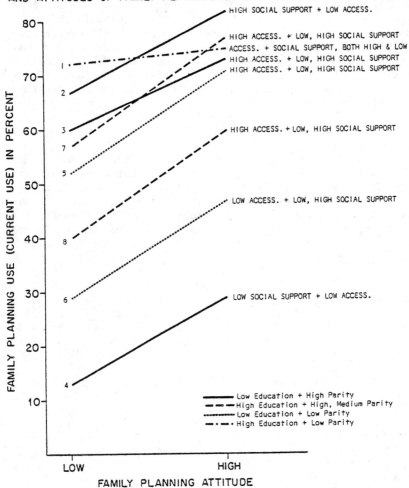

FIGURE 1.
INFLUENCE OF SOCIAL SUPPORT, ACCESSIBILITY,
AND ATTITUDES OF FAMILY PLANNING BY EDUCATION AND PARITY.

tion among respondents with high education and low parity.

The second major finding is that family planning attitude is significantly related with contraception in all four population segments (except those with high education and low parity). In almost all population segments, the difference of the family planning use rates between those with high and low attitudes is over 20 percentage points.

41

Third, social support seems to have the greatest impact amongst those with low education and high parity (graphs 2 and 4). In this segment, even with low accessibility and low attitudes the acceptance rate is about 66 percent; and with favorable attitude, the acceptance is as high as 84 percent.

The major conclusion of the study's results is that a behavior is determined by the combined effects of four factors: (1) cognitive and personal, (2) social support, (3) situational and, (4) accessibility of means or supplies. Consequently, any intervention, to be effective, must carefully evaluate the relative effective of each on a specific population and design the strategy accordingly.

SUMMARY

This paper presents an evaluation of several issues central to marketing and communication strategies for a public health program. These issues are evaluated in terms of the results of a study of the determinants of family planning behavior. Although the data base for the evaluation is limited to fertility behavior, the emphasis has been on the broader implications of this study for marketing and social interventions in public health programs.

The analysis confirms the need for a careful evaluation of the relative impacts of various categories of determinants of the success of such an intervention. Based upon the results of this field study, the paper presents several major implications for a marketing and social intervention according to population segmentation.

This and numerous other studies clearly indicate that behavior is not completely determined by personal preferences and is not always fully rational. Also, regardless of how discomforting the thought may be, we are often influenced by the situational forces. Under the influence of the economic theorists, public health programs in general and family planning programs in particular have developed entire strategies based upon the assumption of the rational man. Liberstein accurately states that those who apply the microeconomic and rational model to explain the contraceptive behavior have "...conjured up the image of every couple having a miniature Wang calculator under their bed on which they work out the balance of the streams of expected benefits and costs... [13, p. 469]". These analysts often ignore the significance of nonrational and situational forces on individual actions. The success of a public health or a marketing program, to a large extent, depends upon these factors; and, a program which is not adequately prepared to deal with such forces may, in spite of its success in "motivating" the people, fail to "change" their behavior.

42

REFERENCES

1. American Marketing Association, Marketing Definitions. Chicago: American Marketing Association, 1960, 15.

2. Callahan, D. "Ethics and Population Limitation," Science, 175 (1972), 487-494.

3. Etzioni, A. "Human Beings Are Not Very Easy To Change After All," Saturday Review, 55 (June 3, 1972), 45-47.

4. Fishbein, M., & Jaccard, J. "Theoretical and Methodological Considerations in the Prediction of Family Planning Intentions and Behavior," Representative Research in Social Psychology, 4 (1973), 37-51.

5. Freedman, R., & Berelson, B. "The Record of Family Planning Programs," Studies in Family Planning, 71 (1976), 1-40.

6. Freedman, R., Hermalin, A.L., and Chang, M.C. "Do Statements About Desired Family Size Predict Fertility? The case of Taiwan," Demography, 12:3 (1975), 407-416.

7. Green, L.W. et al. "Field Experiment Comparing Family Planning Education Programmes Direct at Males and Females," International Journal of Health Education, 16:4 (1973), 242-259.

8. Hochbaum, G.M. "A Critical Assessment of Marketing's Place in Preventive Health Care," Paper presented at the Workshop on Preventive Health Care and Marketing, sponsored by the American Marketing Association, and Blue Cross/Blue Shield of Virginia, Charlottesville, Va., March 27-29, 1977.

9. Hochbaum, G.M. "Public Participation in Medical Screening Programs: A Sociopsychological Study," Public Health Services Publication, 1958, no. 572.

10. Kar, S.B. "Consistency Between Fertility Attitudes and Behavior: A Conceptual Model," Population Studies, forthcoming.

11. Kar, S.B., & Gonzalez-Cerrutti, R. Psychosocial Determinants of Fertility and Contraception: Report of the Baseline Survey 1977, Pan American Health Organization/World Health Organization, forthcoming.

REFERENCES (Cont.)

12. Kasl, S. & Cobb, S. "Health Behavior, Illness Behavior and Sick-role Behavior," Archives of Environmental Health, 12 (February 1966), 246-266, Part I, and 12 (April 1966), 531-541, Part II.

13. Kelman, H.C. "Manipulation of Human Behavior: An Ethical Dilemma for the Social Scientists," In W.G. Bennis (Ed.), The Planning of Change, New York: Holt, Rinehart, and Winston, 1969, 582-595.

14. Liberstein, H. "An Interpretation of the Economic Theory of Fertility: Promising Path or a Blind Alley?," Journal of Economic Literature, 12:2 (1974), 467-479.

15. Marcus, E. "A Study of Unprotected Intercourse Among College Women in Ann Arbor, Michigan, Conducted in 1975," unpublished, Department of Population Planning, University of Michigan, Ann Arbor, Michigan, 1975.

16. Rogers, C.R., & Skinner, B.F. "Some issues concerning the control of human behavior," Science, 124 (1956), 1057-1066.

17. Rosenstock, I.M. "The Health Belief Model and Preventive Health Behavior," In M.H. Becker (Ed.) The Health Belief Model and Personal Health Behavior, New Jersey: Charles B. Slack, Inc., 1974

18. Tell, E. "A Study of Unprotected Intercourse Among College Women in Ann Arbor, Michigan, Conducted in 1975," unpublished, Department of Population Planning, University of Michigan, Ann Arbor, Michigan, 1975.

Special recognition is due to Dr. Ramon Gonzalez-Cerrutti, the co-director of the Venezuela Field Trial project, which provided the data for this paper. The author is indebted to Jeannie Kuo, Kit Frohardt-Lane, and Karen Stanecki for their invaluable assistance with the analysis of the data, and to Professor Richard Landis, who has been particularly helpful with his consultation services for the statistical analysis.

A CONSUMER PERSPECTIVE ON
PREVENTIVE HEALTH CARE SERVICE USAGE*

Philip D. Cooper

THE IMPORTANCE OF ATTITUDES AND SOCIAL INFLUENCES

The study of health service utilization has been saturated
over the years with emphasis on demographic factors as a key to
understanding that behavior. [6] More recently emphasis has
been placed on the role attitudes and social influences play in
the determination of preventive health behavior. [2] Work done
in medical sociology has focused to a great extent on social
influences [1,4,5] as a key determinant of health related behavior (inclusive of health behavior, illness behavior and sick
behavior). The field of social psychology has been ex-
ploring for many years attitudes as they pertain to various behaviors. The field of marketing in its efforts to better understand the way goods are purchased, has suggested that the more
utilitarian a good is, the more important attitudes may be in
the purchase decision. [8] Conversely, the more expressive a
good is - such as clothing which may express one's self image -
the more important normative influences may become in the decision process. It is this marketing perspective that is the
focus of this paper.

It would seem reasonable to expect that services in general may also fall on a continuum from expressive services like
chauffeuring to instrumental services of which preventive health
care services might be an example. If this transference holds,
then it may be reasonable to expect that attitudes would play a
dominant role in the determination of the choice of instrumental services and normative influences would take a dominant
role in the choice of more expressive services. If this were
the case, then the development of communications, educational
programs, etc. may be able to receive guidance in the placement
of emphasis on the attitudinal or normative communication elements with the hopes of increasing the effectiveness of that
communication.

The Health Belief Model has brought together many elements
to help gain a better understanding of "health behavior." One

*The data for this research were developed under a grant by
D.H.E.W. supervised by the Medical Society of Virginia as project #0066 and Employers Mutual Insurance of Wausau.

45

of the more consistently operationalized factors contained in
that model has been the Readiness to Act factor which is composed of two elements – perceived seriousness (PS) of the problem and perceived vulnerability (PV) to the problem. "Readiness to act is defined in terms of the individual's point of
view (or perceptions) about susceptibility (vulnerability) and
seriousness rather than the professional's view of reality."
[7, p. 98 & 99] It is that factor along with the attitudinal
and social normative factors which are the tools used to gain
a better understanding of preventive health care service usage
for this study. An attempt was made to determine the relative
importance of the three factors over time.

THE STUDY DESCRIPTION

The services which were chosen to represent preventive
health care services in general were: the dental exam, general
physical, eye examination, x-ray examination and the Papani-
colaou Smear Test. These were chosen because they were generally readily available, relatively easy to explain, and accessible. More complex and expensive services were not used since
they would have limited the sample population to those who
could afford and/or were familiar with services such as mamography, multiphasic screening, etc.

The population for the initial study was comprised of
female heads of households between the ages of 18 and 64 who
were relatively free to act in a voluntary uninfluenced manner
in seeking preventive health care services. Several screening
questions inquiring about chronic disorders or other matters
such as insurance which might have influenced the use of the
services being studied were necessary to ask.

Data were collected by the use of a proportional stratified
cluster sampling routine with personal interviews conducted by
trained female interviewers. In addition to the screening
questions; demographic data, past service usage data and usage
intention data were also gathered. Data relating to the inter-
viewee's salient reference groups for the services in question
were gathered. Attitudes gathered by pretests generally held
about preventive services, such as "X service saves you time
and money later on" or "X service is painful," were also collected. Data about the key factors of "perceived vulnerability"
and "preceived seriousness" with respect to the diseases or
problem, relating to the services under study were assembled to
develop the "Readiness to Act" factor.

INITIAL STUDY RESULTS

The initial study reported past preventive behavior and

46

intention to use preventive services in the following year. As can be seen in Table 1 (A), attitude was the most important factor followed by readiness to act and the normative factor when past behavior was considered. When intention to use preventive services in the near future became the focus, as demonstrated in Table 1 (B), attitude again takes priority followed by normative and readiness to act factors. The dominance of attitude over the normative factor appears to be consistent with the marketing propositions offered earlier regarding more utilitarian or instrumental services. Whether this relationship is consistent over time becomes an important issue and is explored in the follow up study. It should also be noted that predicability using these three factors increased when the focus became intention to use services as demonstrated by the multiple R.

Another observation is the negative relationship between readiness to act and both intention to use and past usage of preventive services. The label, readiness to act, seems to imply that the higher one is on the scale of readiness to act - that is, if one perceives themselves as being very vulnerable to it - then it seems reasonable to expect a higher intention to use, a higher level of usage and a closer association between intention and usage.

To gain a better understanding of what part readiness to act played, that variable was broken into 4 levels and correlations between intention and usage were analyzed at each level as shown in Figure 1. The findings were that the correlations increased from the lowest level to almost .6 at level 3 then dropped dramatically back when the highest level of readiness to act was reached. This increase at level 3 was accentuated when older respondents were looked at. The correlation reached a level of almost .7. This is demonstrated by the dotted line in Figure 1.

A conclusion which might be drawn is that the readiness to act factor may be acting in a similar manner to fear or perceived risk. That is, beyond a certain optimal level people may be so afraid that behavior no longer may be logical or rational. They may state a high intention to have a test run but refuse to have it actually done because they expect bad results. They may also feel that by actually using the service they may be acknowledging the perceived problem. By not using the service a denial of the perceived problem is demonstrated and this high level of concern may become modified in the mind of the person. One result of this observation is a suggestion to change the label of this factor in the Health Belief Model from readiness to act to "Level of Concern" which allows for the

Table 1 (A)

Factor Importance for
Past Usage of Preventive Services (PPB)
(N=405, DF=3,401)

| | Study Factors | | |
	Attitude	Normative	Readiness to Act
Factor Entry (stepwise regression)	1	3	2
F level	10.6*	6.0*	9.2*
Beta	.17	.13	−.15
Multiple R	.215	.278	.252
R	.215	.026	.037

*significant at or beyond the .05 level

Table 1 (B)

Factor Importance for
Intention to Use Preventive Services (PBI)
(N=405, DF=3,401)

| | Study Factors | | |
	Attitude	Normative	Readiness to Act
Factor Entry (stepwise regression)	1	2	3
F level	26.7*	12.7*	.098
Betas	.26	.18	−.015
Multiple R	.329	.368	.369
R	.329	.039	.001

*significant at or beyond the .05 level

possibility for consideration of an optimum level not the highest level to show the most consistency.

FIGURE 1

CORRELATIONS BETWEEN USAGE AND USAGE INTENTION

BASED ON CATEGORIES OF READINESS TO ACT (PV) (PS)

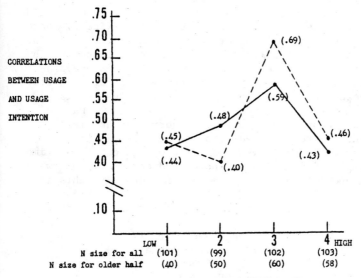

FOUR CATEGORIES OF READINESS TO ACT

—————— Correlations for entire sample (N= 405)

— — — — Correlations for only the older half of the sample (N= 208)

(Note: All correlations are significant at the .01 level or better)

FOLLOW UP STUDY RESULTS

A mail follow up study and a control group study was conducted after about one year. The purpose of the control group was to provide a benchmark against which to determine if, as a result of the initial interview about preventive health care, the original respondents were sensitized to the use of these services. Except for the use of x-ray examinations for preventive purposes, the original respondents did not demonstrate higher usage of the services. Because of attrition in the original sample, the more mobile younger and more highly educated were reduced in representation leaving an older population which may be more prone to use those services and perhaps less aware of the controversy involved in the use of x-ray.

49

The response rate for the follow up group was 76% which provided a sufficient sample size to work with. Additional
screening questions were used to account for changes in health
status and other matters which might affect the usage of the
services.

The results of the study, as shown in Table 2, demonstrate
that the relationship between attitudes and normative factors
is apparently stable over the time of the study. Attitude
again is more important than the normative factor in predicting
actual preventive usage. The difference is significant. Here
again we see the "level of concern" or readiness to act factor
contributing to predictability but in an inverse manner which
is consistent with the previous measures. There is one dis-
turbing observation and that is the overall level of predictability of these measures dropped from the previous levels.
This problem may stem from a weakness of the study. Due to
time, money and convenience, attitude, normative and level of
concern measures were gathered at only one point in time,
whereas, behavior measures were gathered over a period of time.
This would imply that attitudes, norms and concern levels were
expected to be consistent over time. Unfortunately, this is

Table 2

Factor Importance for
Actual Preventive Service Usage (APB)
Follow-up Study
(N=268, DF=3,264)

| | | Study Factor | |
	Attitude	Normative	Readiness to Act
Factor Entry (stepwise regression)	1	3	2
F level	7.0*	.1	1.6
Beta	.16	.02	-.08
Multiple R	.160	.178	.177
R	.16	.001	.017

*significant at or beyond the .05 level

not the case. Had these changes been able to be taken into account, the level of predictability may have remained at a more consistent level with the previous measures.

DISCUSSION

One resultant element of the analysis is a guideline that might be established concerning the development of communications about preventive services in general or at least the set of services used for this study. Based on the consistency of attitude's enduring importance over the normative factor, it would seem reasonable to stress attitudinal factors in the program development and communications aimed at increasing the useage of preventive care. This would be especially true when there is a limited amount of time during which to present material. A 30 second radio or T.V. spot commercial or public service announcement would be an example.

Another outcome of the study might be the suggestion to develop a cautious approach to the design of communication aimed at increasing a person's perceptions about the seriousness and vulnerability to a disease. If the objective of the communication is to increase usage of preventive services, then increasing a person's perceptions to the highest level of concern may actually reduce usage. Perhaps the development of a benchmark based on public (or target market) levels of concern might provide guidelines which may acutally dictate the development of a program to reduce the public's level to a more optimal action oriented level.

REFERENCES

1. Anderson, R. & F. F. Newman. "Societal and Individual Determinants of Medical Care Utilization in the United States," Milbank Memorial Fund Quarterly, 51 (Winter 1973), pp. 95-124.

2. Becker, M. H. (Ed.) "The Health Belief Model and Personal Health Behavior," Health Education Monographs, 2 (Winter 1974).

3. Cooper, P. D. A Marketing Investigation of Preventive Health Care Service Usage, Final Report for Project #0066, DHEW, DRMP, Medical Society of Virginia, October 1977.

4. Glasser, M. A. "A Study of the Public's Acceptance of the Salk Vaccine Program, American Journal of Public Health, 48 (February 1958), pp. 141-146.

REFERENCES (Cont.)

5. Koos, E. The Health of Regionville, New York: Hafner, 1954.

6. McKinlay, J. B. "Some Approaches and Problems in the Study of the Use of Services -- An Overview." Journal of Health and Social Behavior, 13 (June 1972), pp. 115-152.

7. Rosenstock, I. M., "Why People Use Health Services," Milbank Memorial Fund Quarterly, 44 (July 1966, part 2), pp. 94-127.

8. Wilson, D., H. L. Mathews and J. Harvey. "An Empirical Test of the Fishbein Behavioral Intention Model," Journal of Consumer Research, 1 (March 1975), pp. 39-48.

AN OVERVIEW OF APPROACHES TO KNOWLEDGE OF
PREVENTIVE HEALTH CARE BEHAVIOR

Charles O. Crawford

After the presentations it was noted that the dissatisfaction with the KAB or KAP model derives not so much from the nature of the data collected but the way the analysis is done. If the analysis is done in much greater detail, as Kar had done his, much more could be derived from already existing data rather than go out and collect more data.

Godfrey Hochbaum (who shared in the development of the Health Belief Model) observed that, in the health belief model, perceived seriousness and perceived susceptibility were not really meant to be part of "readiness to act" as it might be interpreted from the literature. "Readiness to act" was meant more to be part of the cue element of the health belief model. Dr. Hochbaum commented on some of the findings which Cooper found regarding the curvilinear relationship on level of concern factor in which the persons with the highest level of concern had lower levels of actual and intended usage than did those with lower levels of concern. Dr. Hochbaum noted that in his work with use of X-rays as a preventive measure for tuberculosis, those who were truly worried had already gone to their physician and thus did not use the X-ray technique as much. He stressed that those who were quite sure that they were O.K. and had no signs or symptoms of lung disease were like a college student--all set to take the test. Dr. Hochbaum also noted the importance of social normative factor in his work. When individuals came in groups, the health belief model did not explain use of the X-ray. However, the health belief model did provide explanatory power when individuals came by themselves. He said this suggested the importance of considering social support in health behavior.

It was observed that subjective accessibility as presented by Kar was very important and that this represented an attribute of the quality of service delivered. It represented an attempt to improve the product offered.

Dr. Kar reviewed with workshop participants some of the findings obtained when path analysis was applied to his data on family planning. Some of the best results on adoption of family planning were obtained when the variables of access and social support were allowed through the attitude variable rather than relate them directly to adoption of preventive health behavior.

53

III

SPECIAL TOPICS IN PREVENTIVE HEALTH CARE MARKETING

An interesting series of concurrent discussions comprised this part of the workshop. Included are reviews of such discussions as the role of advertising in preventive health care, the ethics of such advertising, the acceptability of marketing in the preventive health care arena, discussion on the utilization of incentives to affect preventive health care service usage, and considerations of the place of consumer research in guiding preventive health policies.

ADVERTISING PREVENTIVE HEALTH CARE: INFORMATIONAL, PERSUASIVE, ETHICAL?

Mark Moriarty

GENERAL ISSUES

A problem of considerable concern is the definition of preventive health care. The task advertising has to perform will vary substantially depending on the meaning attached to the term. If, for instance, preventive services are advertised which involve the delivery of specific services, tangible measures of demand stimulation effectiveness can be used to monitor campaign results. If, however, advertising campaigns are undertaken to promote long-run life style changes (i.e., reduction of alcohol and cigarette consumption), the task is unique in that people are asked to <u>give up habits</u>. In these situations, intermediate and less tangible (communications) performance measures may have to be employed to measure campaign results in lieu of measuring the long-run results.

A second and somewhat related problem is the setting of advertising priorities. Some would argue that the various organizations concerned with promoting preventive health should attempt to change health behavior where the short run results are tangible. Certainly advertising expenditure allocations which produce tangible results would more easily be justified. Others would view this approach as myopic and inconsequential to the long-run goal of promoting changes in habits which result in more healthful life styles. The present state of knowledge concerning advertising's effectiveness over the substantial time periods required to change health habits will probably not allow definitive statements to be made concerning priorities. These judgements will have to be made by the organizations involved and are very likely to be strongly affected by situation-specific conditions confronting these organizations.

A third issue of concern is who will pay for preventive health care advertising programs. The general feeling is that since the consumer is the one to reap the benefits, he should be the one to pay the bill. A unique feature of many organizations promoting preventive health care is that they are often dependent on several groups of "publics" which have a vested interest in their performance. Dependence on multiple groups for support sometimes leads to conflicts over goals and policies and when these goals are in conflict, support is on occasion withdrawn. On a macro level, there is an issue of who has the organizational responsibility for advertising preventive health care. Should it be with government, the medical community, or perhaps philanthropic organizations? An obvious premise to a rational program for promoting preventive care should be the determination of organizational responsibility so that the public is exposed to a uniform and coherent message.

INFORMATIONAL ISSUES

The informational content of preventive health care advertising seems to be the paramount issue in view of the fact that preventive care (in most but not all of its forms) appears to involve new behaviors or a modification of existing behavior. New or innovative behavior typically is preceded by an individual decision process which leads to adoption of the behavior. The individual in the initial stages of the adoption process requires from the source of the innovation (the organization promoting the preventive health measure) extensive information in order to made a decision. Specifically, the information should provide (a) awareness of where services are available, (b) awareness of what services are available, (c) awareness of the cost of services to the individual if any, (d) awareness of the opportunity cost for not using the service, and (e) awareness of how to use the service. If the organization is promoting a specific health care practice rather than a service, the information in the advertising should indicate where the individual can receive more extensive and detailed (printed) information to aid in deciding whether or not to adopt the practice.

A related issue concerns the state of information that different target audiences have with respect to preventive health care practices or services. Organizations advertising preventive health should recognize that different target audiences are going to be at different stages in the adoption process, and these stages require different advertising strategies. Prior knowledge of these differences is of significant importance in determining appropriate strategies.

Examples cited in the session suggest that, for those advertised preventive services which promote actions that can be immediately taken and have immediate results, the response is quite strong in terms of patient demand. A political financial and ethical question is whether or not the health care delivery mechanism can meet the anticipated demand. This appears to be a research question involving the measurement of demand. For those long run lifestyle changes (proper diet, exercises, etc.) the persuasive effectiveness of advertising is much more questionable. The problem centers on the measurement of long run effectiveness, especially the relationship between future health outcomes in the population and current preventive health care advertising campaigns.

Another issue involving persuasion and competition is the apparently conflicting messages which emanate from different media sources and promote behavior which conflict with preventive behaviors (smoking vs. non-smoking). The results of such competition is often a confused public. Coherent national policies which clearly delineate advertising's role are needed.

ETHICAL ISSUES

Ethical issues of advertising seem to be raised primarily by the medical care providers. Doctors appear to believe that advertising will foster competition and somehow competition among health care professionals for patients is counterproductive to good health care practice. Some session members expressed the view that this position was meant to limit competition and insure healthy fees for services rather than for altrusic motives related to quality of care. Some session members also expressed the view that non-profit institutions (such as hospitals) which provide preventive services may feel uncomfortable with advertising. The fear apparently is that the community will not look favorably on the institution if it uses operating funds to promote preventive services when such promotion raises patient fees for services. However, it should be pointed out that this relationship will not necessarily occur if excess capacity exists. In this case additional revenue will reduce fees since it should make at least a marginal contribution to fixed costs.

In an attempt to clarify ethical questions related to advertising, an important distinction to be made is between service vs. non-service advertising such as between a pap smear test (a specific test requiring a fee) and advertising of seat belt usage (no fee or service rendered by an institution). That is, if the advertising is meant to stimulate demand for specific services, the medical community seems to be more concerned with

56

the ethics of the advertising. If general preventive health
procedures are advertised, there seems to be no ethical problem.

The final issue to be raised is that of advertising claims.
Preventive health care behavior in some cases has only long run
and uncertain outcomes for the individual. Advertising claims
of a more healthy life associated with specific changes in behavior will have to be documented to satisfy the present federal
guidelines of the FTC. It does appear that present agencies
regulating advertising will be sufficient to handle the advertising of preventive health care. No new agencies appear needed
to handle the uniquenesses of this form of advertising.

IS MARKETING TOO STIGMATIZED TO
BE EFFECTIVELY ACCEPTED IN PREVENTIVE
HEALTH CARE

Robert M. Chamberlain

After considerable discussion the conclusion is that marketing is probably not too stigmatized to be an effective tool in preventive health care. In fact, a number of marketing techniques such as market segmentation, consumer decision-making research, and product image-making are currently employed in public health education. Health education usually seeks to sell health practices rather than merely inform the public. Hence it is more than education in the narrow sense, because it promotes a particular conclusion desired by the health educator. If marketing techniques are called by other names and employed successfully by public health educators we must conclude that such stigma that exists is associated with the marketing discipline rather than with the tools of marketing. The ideological separation of the commerce/business sector and the helping professions has perhaps stigmatized the image of the marketing discipline in the eyes of the traditional physician.

The type of large health organization which may be in best position to apply a forthright marketing approach is likely to be dominated by medical administrators who are not physicians and by physicians who are oriented to broad-scale community preventive medicine. These individuals are less directed by the requirements of acute disease intervention and have more self-interest in preventive practices. Their organizations are HMO's, industrial practices, and public health settings; all of which benefit economically by keeping their clientele healthy. Marketing holds for them, an opportunity to achieve certain objectives and there is little reason to believe that stigma will stand in the way. Our concern should be that marketing will not be equipped to fulfill the expectations of the health professionals. Such expectations may be exaggerated beyond the capabilities of marketing practitioners. The marketer who achieves a 15 percent change in consumer behavior will very likely be viewed as a failure by health professionals expecting 99 percent compliance. Marketing practitioners must be aware of this danger and not oversell their capabilities in the health care arena.

UTILIZATION OF INCENTIVES TO AFFECT
PREVENTIVE HEALTH CARE SERVICE USAGE

Reed Morton

In the commercial sector, incentives are a familiar technique for promoting product consumption. If incentives are to assume a role in promoting preventive health care, it first is necessary to understand the nature and limits of this approach to influencing consumption behavior.

Incentives are intended as positive additions to the usual benefits of consumption. As such, they differ from measures to facilitate consumption or enhance accessibility which aim to remove barriers or other "negative benefits" involved in consummating exchanges. It's also necessary to distinguish incentives from the broader notion of reinforcement. Incentives are, in the present situation, inducements to emit a desired preventive health behavior. They are provided or administered before the behavior occurs. Like an incentive, reinforcement may be gratifying--if positive--but, as part of a learning situation, it is a reward provided only after the desired behavior has occurred.

Incentives have the important job of bringing people to what may be their first contact with preventive health care. The marketer's specialty is identifying values in exchanges and that specialized knowledge obviously needs some application in preventive health care situations.

A LACK OF MANY EXAMPLES

Few examples of preventive health incentives were apparent in the discussion group's experience. Offering a service (an X-ray or another screening measure) free is an obvious type of incentive. Another suggestion was the practice of extending compensatory leave time to federal employees who become blood donors. If any participant in the health sector could be expected to employ incentives, insurers seemed most appropriate. One hope was that a Wausau-type approach might develop--working with beneficiaries to identify risks and adopt preventive measures. To encourage screening and early treatment, an insurer might pay the cost of screenings which detect a symptom, if the patient obtained treatment for the condition immediately. The patient who postponed treatment would pay for the screening tests.

59

Given so few empirical examples of incentives for preventive health care, a more conceptual focus becomes appropriate. A consensus favoring multifaceted approaches to offering inducements evolved. One aspect of this varied approach related to the locus of incentivization. Three socializing agents were considered: schools, parents, and peers.

A problem connected with any school-based strategy is the increasing concern with inadequate performance in the traditional and basic school functions--reading, writing, arithmetic. Many would resist attempts to lodge another responsibility on educators already besieged with "educationally related" programs. Parents were recognized as already having a role in providing or inducing preventive care for children. Unfortunately, too few seem to perform as hoped. A suggested solution would incentivize the parental role as the first step to reaching children's behavior.

The role of peers in shaping behavior, particularly among adolescents, presents a challenge. Peer regard frequently motivates smoking behavior. Not only would incentives be required to secure initiation of non-smoking behavior, additional reinforcers would be necessary to maintain the new health practice. If status among peers attached to stopping smoking and beginning and continuing an exercise program, the challenge would be reduced.

The participants in the discussion group examined their own incentives for adopting health enhancing behavior, and identified the recognition of a statistical likelihood of better health, longer life and the more subjective benefit of feeling better. Not one of the benefits might seem especially persuasive to a teenage smoker enjoying status among relevant peers. Furthermore, reasons were identified and found for not adopting healthier practices valid for adolescents, too. There were no incentives to change nor were negative sanctions applied while the behaviors continued.

CONCLUSION

In conclusion, initial attention might address environmental disincentives for preventive health: larger than necessary restaurant portions, one floor elevator trips, riding school buses. As emphasis shifts to using incentives, providing inducements which reward partial compliance may become an important strategy.

THE PLACE OF CONSUMER RESEARCH IN GUIDING
PREVENTIVE HEALTH POLICIES

Robert W. Denniston

PREVENTIVE HEALTH POLICIES

Prior to the topic discussion, there was comment about the current state of affairs relating to preventive health policies. Several participants noted that no one group or sector of society presently intends to determine what preventive health activities should exist and then to plan and direct such activities. The federal government has only recently begun to think in terms of a national focus on preventive health. State governments now are beginning to realize the importance of preventive health as they are taking on the financial burden of delivery of health care. The private sector is just beginning to make an effort to market products or services that effect preventive health care.

WHO SHOULD DO CONSUMER RESEARCH?

The question of who should be doing consumer research arose from the earlier question of who is involved in preventive health policies. Several participants pointed out that it does not make much difference as long as reputable organizations were doing the research and findings were shared. The funding of such research, a critical issue, was discussed briefly, with the comment that bias due to source of funding is common but usually quite apparent, not insidious. Ideally, research without such bias is desirable, but difficult to obtain.

WHEN SHOULD RESEARCH BE DONE?

More important than who is doing the research is the question of when. Research must be done as health policies are being considered, not after the policy is decided and the program is underway. Participants' anecdotal information supported the observation that too often research is done after policies are decided, not at a time when the policies are being formulated. Research must be an integral part of policy making and the planning process.

Furthermore, research must be used, not ignored. Often, appropriate research was conducted but the results were ignored when the findings were inconsistent with an expedient political point of view. The political process in many instances determines preventive health policies more often than good research,

61

largely because of the role of government in determining policies. Research can be most useful at the policy formulation stage by helping to determine the feasibility and cost-effectiveness of proposed policies.

The timeliness of research is a key factor. The lengthy process of getting research underway and completed can be a problem, particularly when using government-collected data. The national health survey, for example, takes two and one-half years to collect and analyze information about respondents, and yet the availability of certain kinds of attitudinal questions to be asked still is quite limited. To be effective consumer research should be early, prominent and continuous.

CONSUMER RESEARCH PURPOSES

In the commercial world, consumer research generally is done for two reasons: (1) to help shape the product or service, and (2) to determine how the product or service should be promoted. In the preventive health field, all too often the shape of the product or service has already been decided, by someone else such as doctors or government. The swine flu immunization program is a good example. The question was not how to shape the product (that had been decided scientifically and politically) but how to promote the product. Consumer research might have told us something about attitudes relating to the seriousness of flu in the public's estimation, about attitudes towards the federal government, about any program calling itself "100 per cent voluntary." Such research might have resulted in a more successful program.

Preventing such research in this case, however, were bureaucratic obstacles which not only precluded adequate consumer research but raised new problems as well. For example, issuing a contract to develop promotional materials or obtaining approval from the Office of Management and Budget on a survey questionnaire, (normally necessary steps in a program of this magnitude), would have taken months of additional delay.

NATIONAL HEALTH POLICIES

Rather than a single national policy or a series of policies in preventive health set by the government, there is in reality a mosaic of policies, set by federal and state governments, by voluntary agencies, by health care professionals' associations, by businesses and universities and private concerns, often at a fragmented, categorical level. This vigorous mosaic is a source of great strength, but long range planning is necessary, and the federal government should take the initiative and the responsibility for this by conducting the kind of research that would make such planning possible.

An example of such research leading to a specific program is the smoking and health survey conducted periodically. Such research, it was agreed, should be shared with appropriate voluntary and other organizations to aid them in their planning efforts. The National High Blood Pressure Education Program was given as an example of how government can make use of data available through consumer research and can plan long range efforts to work with voluntary and private organizations in such a way that a definite focus is achieved and the resulting coordination is effective in creating a truly national program.

Too often, short range goals and high-yield programs are set up to show an immediate pay off for efforts and money invested. Longer-range planning, however, could permit more consequential results, although not immediately measurable. Again, it was agreed that government ought to play a role in defining what long-range planning in preventive health is possible by conducting consumer research that would lead to realistic and effective policy-making.

IV.

PERCEPTIONS OF PROBLEMS AND LIMITATIONS OF
PREVENTIVE HEALTH CARE AND MARKETING

An interesting segment of the workshop centered on four concurrent panel discussions on perceptions of problems and limitations of preventive health care and marketing. Each panel consisted of one representative from academics, government and the practitioners, plus four or five other participants. The panels and their topics included

A. From The Viewpoint of Government

B. From The Academic View

C. From The Practitioners View

D. Problems and Limitations: Summary Comments

IV. A. FROM THE VIEWPOINT OF GOVERNMENT

Included here are papers treating perceptions of problems and limitations of preventive health care and marketing from a governmental viewpoint. Papers by William A. Flexner, Patricia Q. Schoeni and Graham W. Ward comprise this section.

BY CHOICE A LIMITED GOVERNMENT ROLE

William A. Flexner

While the federal government could stimulate an increase in the use of marketing concepts and techniques throughout the health field, to date it has chosen a more limited role. There are at least three reasons for this:

-- a narrow interpretation of the role of marketing in health care;

-- deference to the private sector; and

-- questions of accountability and liability.

CONCEPTS OF PREVENTIVE HEALTH CARE

Preventive health care begins with individual behavior and expands outward to include, among other things, the use of pre-

64

ventive health services. (There are also many social and environmental actions which have an impact on the health of individuals. However, because such actions do not require individual behavior to be effective, they are omitted from this discussion.) Considered in the light of individual behavior, preventive health care refers to <u>actions taken by individuals to
decrease the likelihood or risk of illness, disease or injury</u>.
These actions include:

-- such personal habits as eating, smoking and exercise;

-- the purchase of such things as nutritious foods, "safe"
   consumer products, and contraceptives; and

-- the use of such preventive health services as immunizations, physical examinations, screening programs, and
   family planning.

A KEY PROBLEM IN PREVENTIVE HEALTH CARE

One of the major reasons that preventive health care has a
relatively low priority among consumers is that all concerned
entities -- marketers, government officials, and health practitioners -- have placed too much emphasis on the product -- that
is, the services and messages related to preventive health --
and not enough on the intended recipients of the product -- the
consumers, their motivations, and the benefits that attract them
to certain behaviors. Instead of focusing on alternative behaviors related to obesity in order to match certain individuals
with specific behavior responses, diets or some other "global"
response are featured. No wonder it is not very effective.

This problem is similar to the marketing dilemna of whether
to adopt a product or consumer orientation. The orientation
ultimately adopted says a lot about the marketing activities
that will be considered relevant for implementation.

PRODUCT VS. CONSUMER ORIENTATION IN
PREVENTIVE HEALTH CARE MARKETING

A good example of the problem just cited is what the writer interprets to be the health field's view towards marketing.
In this view, marketing means promotion -- advertising and
health education -- and has little relationship to product or
service design, price, and place. By equating marketing with
only one of the four Ps -- promotion -- the health field is
demonstrating that its primary orientation is generally toward
the product (usually defined in technical-medical terms) and not
the consumer. Were it otherwise, marketing concepts and techniques would be considered relevant to preventive health care

in the following areas:

-- Product: Design and development of consumer-responsive preventive health care goods, services, or ideas

-- Price: Consideration of direct costs, opportunity costs, incentives, trade-offs related to preventive health behaviors

-- Promotion: Use of personal and impersonal communication to associate benefits with goods, services, or ideas and to attract consumers to their use

-- Place: Focus on ease of access to intended or desired preventive health behaviors -- access refers to both physical and psychological space

In short, to be effective, preventive health care marketing -- just like commercial and industrial marketing -- must encompass all four of the controllable marketing variables.

PRODUCTS AND BRANDS IN PREVENTIVE HEALTH CARE: AN EXAMPLE

The above reference to pushing "global" responses to individual-specific behaviors highlights another aspect of marketing that has important implications in preventive health care. This is the distinction between the product class and the brand. An example from the field of family planning illustrates the point:

Promotion of the use of family planning services has traditionally focused on a group of alternative behaviors as a whole. This grouping of behaviors is equivalent to marketing's product class. The resulting messages include references to "responsible parenthood" and "family welfare" or to "family planning" as in the following example which comes from a study carried out in 1971, where radio and television ads were used to recruit family planning service consumers to clinics in several U. S. cities. [1]

ANNCR: Having a baby isn't easy. That's why for a healthy mother and a healthy child, it's always best to allow time between births. And by spacing your children, you'll be able to give them the love and attention they need. Being a good parent takes time and love and planning.

Family Planning, for couples who want children . . . later.

66

LOCAL ANNCR: For information, call ....

When the ad campaign failed to produce an increase in demand
for services, one of the conclusions made by the investigators
was that the message had to be more specific regarding the fertility control method being advocated. Given the preliminary
results of a followup study where the focus of the campaign was
on only one technique of fertility control -- vasectomy -- this
conclusion appears to have been justified: the demand for vasectomy services increased simultaneously with the airing of
vasectomy-specific radio ads in two cities, while the demand was
increasing in the control city. [2] Focus on vasectomy, as in
this example, is equivalent to a marketing focus at the brand
level.

MARKETING AND PREVENTIVE HEALTH CARE: BY CHOICE A LIMITED GOVERNMENT ROLE

Having suggested some problems in preventive health care
and marketing, what has been the federal government's role?
And, what are the prospects for the future?

Traditionally, the federal government has maintained a passive involvement in the provision of preventive health services.
For the most part, such services have been seen as the function
of the private sector, with deference paid thereto. Nonethe-
less, the government has participated actively in preventive
health care through regulations to assure public safety and
through the allocation of financial resources to affect the distribution and use of existing health resources, and to stimulate the design and delivery of new health resources. Finally,
the government has attempted to promote preventive health behavior, but in so doing has focused primarily on what is described as the product class, and only seldomly at the brand
level.

It is the importance of focusing on brands in the context
of the four Ps that promote the following conclusions about the
role of government in marketing and preventive health care:

-- For marketing to be effective, it must focus on specific brands

-- To focus on specific brands of goods, services or ideas
   requires a willingness to accept the responsibility
   and liability for failure.

-- Except in unusual circumstances (swine flu vaccines),
   the government defers to the private sector for the provision of specific brands of goods, services, or ideas,

and is reluctant to accept the liability for them

-- Thus the government is unlikely to use marketing in the field of preventive health care

-- Furthermore, because the government appears to interpret marketing narrowly as promotion, it is not likely to use its financial resources to stimulate a broader use of marketing concepts and techniques in the private sector

CONCLUSION

Some things that need to be done in marketing and preventive health care are suggested in conclusion.

First, a better description of the possible multiple applications of marketing concepts and techniques in preventive health care is needed; applications that involve each of the four Ps, not just one of them as is now the case.

Second, from a marketing -- not a health -- point of view, considerably more information is needed about the behavior of individuals vis-a-vis preventive health. This would involve studies which focus on the behavioral choices that consumers make which affect their health negatively and positively, and the motivations behind those choices.

Finally, if the government is expected to use its resources to stimulate a broader use of marketing concepts and techniques in preventive health care, then individuals who have commercial experience in marketing management must be brought into the government at a sufficiently high level to have an impact on policies and programs in marketing terms.

REFERENCES

1. J. Richard Udry, et al., The Media and Family Planning. Cambridge: Ballinger, 1974, p. 67.

2. Winfield Best, et al., "A Test of Advertising Vasectomy on Radio." Chapel Hill, NC: Carolina Population Center, 1977, (in draft).

FROM THE FEDERAL PERSPECTIVE

Patricia Q. Schoeni

There is little argument about the value of preventive health care. In recent years, it has become more evident that only by preventing disease from occurring, rather than treating it later, can we hope to achieve any major improvement in the Nation's health.

The problem of disease prevention itself has changed radically since 1900 when pneumonia, influenza, and tuberculosis were among the leading causes of death. Today, heart disease, cancer, accidents and mental illness have taken their place. The scourge of communicable diseases has been supplanted by that of chronic diseases in the last half of this century. In 1972, an estimated 26 million people were disabled by chronic diseases.

A distinctive feature of many of the chronic conditions, however, is that they are caused by factors, such as individual behavior and the environment, that are not susceptible to direct medical intervention. Cigarette smoking, for example, is considered to be primarily responsible for a large number of diseases afflicting society, from lung cancer and heart disease to chronic bronchitis. But it is also a major social, economic, cultural and psychological phenomenon. Nor can the ever-increasing chemical contamination of our water, air, and food be viewed solely from a medical perspective. There is much greater recognition today that the kinds and amounts of food and liquor we consume and the style of living in our sedentary society are major contributing factors to the development of chronic illness, and that to change these patterns of behavior requires the active involvement of the individual.

DISEASE CONTROL

Many diseases are no longer inexplicable events beyond man's control. An overwhelming proportion of them are caused by man and his institutions and can be controlled by man. Thus, an important component of preventive medicine is the education of individuals to the underlying causes of disease and how they can reduce the chances of becoming subject to many of those chronic conditions. Over the next several years, all health programs of The Department of Health, Education and Welfare will seek ways to concentrate their energies and talent on attacking the causes of disease and on helping people and communities to take direct responsibility for protecting their own health.

69

There is, however, some argument about the subject and substance of the preventive health care messages. There is even more argument about who is best able to carry those messages to the public. The messages usually center around the following areas:

1) Information about personal practices that affect health, such as personal cleanliness, safety measures, exercise, smoking, alcohol and drug use and eating habits;

2) Use of appropriate health services, such as Emergency Medical Services systems, recognition of signs and symptoms requiring immediate attention, and the availability of special clinics and services;

3) Special areas of concern, such as immunization, venereal disease, genetic counseling, family planning and pre- and post-natal care; and

4) Management of chronic illness to prevent further break- down, such as taking prescribed medication and under- going necessary rehabilitation procedures.

MARKETING HEALTH CARE MESSAGES

But who should market these messages? On the individual level, is it the physician, the professional health educator, the community leader or the community member who is best able to carry the message? And on the organizational level, is it the local government agencies, the voluntary associations, the schools, the State Health Departments or the Federal Government who should have the primary responsibility for promoting pre- ventive health care? If the Federal Government has a role in marketing prevention, what is that role and how effectively can it be carried out?

One of the basic problems in marketing prevention is the traditional public orientation toward cure of illness rather than maintenance of health. We have made some progress in pub- lic reorientation in this regard, but we still have a good dis- tance to go. And, this factor obviously makes preventive health care more difficult to market than most products or services.

Those marketing efforts that the Federal Government has undertaken have had varying degrees of success--or failure. Some of those efforts worked exceptionally well. Such was the case with the polio vaccine campaign. Others produced results which, if not those that were expected, were nevertheless posi- tive, such as the anti-smoking effort. While still others were disastrous, such as in the area of drug abuse.

When the Federal Government markets preventive health care activities, there exists certain restraints that can limit success. These restraints include political and public pressures, dilution of the message to achieve appropriateness and/or universality and prohibitions against paid advertising time or space.

CONCLUSION

In light of these and other restraints, should the Federal Government be marketing preventive health care? If the answer is "no," then who should? If the answer is "yes," then how can the adverse effects of these restraints be minimized? And if the answer is "sometimes," what are the areas in which the Federal Government should assume responsibility?

If these questions are answered--which will not be a simple task--society will be closer to answering the questions, "Can preventive health care be effectively marketed, and, if so, how?"

THE ROLE OF ECONOMICS, UTILIZATION
AND UNCERTAINTY

Graham W. Ward

PROLOGUE

Any discussion of preventive health care and marketing and limitations of these efforts should, most reasonably, start with an operating definition of what these terms are. Preventive health care encompasses a broad field requiring specific actions on the part of health care consumers and providers alike which are designed, not only to avoid disease, but also to achieve an optimum health status. Prevention of disease is a concept with little ambiguity. Achieving optimum health is quite another issue. Operationally, it would seem reasonable to define health as the capability of achieving one's personal goals under conditions which minimize adverse stress and which maximize those kinds of stresses which contribute positively to goal achievement. Given these few brief assumptions, it becomes immediately apparent that health is not the same for each individual, and that one of the current major concerns of the American public, stress, must also be defined on an individual basis.

Given this prologue, it is evident that marketing must be described in the same broad terms as being actions by others intended to persuade or motivate an individual to adopt certain specific actions which are generally accepted by society as being beneficial and providing for the majority of individuals an increased probability of achieving individual goals.

THE ECONOMIC VIEWPOINT

Because the most broadly held concept of marketing involves the inducement of consumers to make investments, it seems reasonable to begin the discussion from an economic viewpoint. Educators, health care providers, economists and marketing people, while using quite different jargon in their respective fields, share a basic commonality of interest. Few participants of this conference would take exception to the statement that the actions of all these various professionals focus on changing the actions or behavior of people and upon the factors which influence people's actions. Economics is not just a dollars and cents science, but also a behavioral science examining how resources are developed, exchanged and consumed -- resources such as time, materials, and knowledge. Development, exchange and consumption are behaviorist. The dollars and cents comes in as a means of providing a convenient standard unit for expressing the diversity

72

of resources involved. The means of assessing the units -- value setting -- is a key human behavior. In this writer's view, Machiavelli, Sigmond Freud, John Maynard Keynes, Albert Lasker or you or I, are all behavioral scientists. They and we differ only in the terms used to describe behavior.

The relationship of economics and behavioral sciences can be seen most clearly by considering motivational theory. For the purposes of discussion, a grossly over-simplified model is used. Generally speaking, before an individual engages in any specific activity or behavior, four steps must occur - usually in the following sequence. 1.) the individual must know or be aware that the particular behavior or activity is among the options from which he can choose. 2.) he must be able to understand the behavior. By understanding, he must be able to place it in perspective within his own life space and relate it to others in his own vocabulary. 3.) he must possess the capability to perform the behavior. In other words, there must be neither physical nor social barriers to his action that are insurmountable with the resources at his command. 4.) the individual must see some value or payoff in a particular behavior which is greater than the value or payoff he perceives in an alternate course of action. These four steps, whether taken consciously or without thought, are those which take us down every path of life including the paths leading into, through and out of the economist's so-called market place.

CONSUMER HEALTH CARE UTILIZATION

It may be useful, at this point, to examine some of the economic reasons why consumers use or do not use health care resources. In examining consumer behavior relative to the seeking of health care services, Bailey [1] divides these services into three categories: emergency or life-threatening care needs, ordinary curative and restorative care and preventive care. His description of consumer behavior is one you might well predict. In life-threatening situations, neither price nor the consumers income have much effect on the demand for this type of care. For ordinary curative care, however, the demand closely resembles that for any commodity in the open market. If the price is high or the consumer's income is low, the demand is less. If the price is low or the consumer's income is high, then demand increases. For preventive services Bailey states, "unless the price is lowered almost to or at zero, it is doubtful that demand for these services can be stimulated through the regular market (price) incentives." He further asserts that increasing the consumption of preventive services would require a substantial educational effort and improvement in the techniques of practice to reduce the uncertainty attached to the value of such services. Consumer uncertainty

is a key term that also merits a brief definition. To quote
Bailey again, "if the consumer is rational, he will not buy
preventive health services unless he can be convinced that the
. . . utility of the service will exceed the . . . utility (of)
other goods and services. There is little opportunity to measure the size of the risk that is undertaken by failure to purchase the service. The data did not exist in most instances.
Thus, the purchase of preventive services presents a case of
consumption under a high degree of uncertainty leading to what
appears to be a rational decision on the part of consumers: a
decision not to purchase such services."

LIMITATIONS

To discuss the limitations of preventive health care and
marketing, each is viewed in terms of the four steps in the
simplified model presented earlier. For those interested in a
more complex approach, examination of the Health Belief Model
as modified by Marshall Becker is recommended (Figure #1). The
first step is awareness on the part of the individual that a
given preventive action is an option available to him; that he
is aware that that action possibility exists among his range of
options. In terms of preventive health care, this implies that
a state-of-the-art has been reached which permits us to say that
a given action will have a predictable health outcome. Taking
hypertension as an example, in the early 1960's drugs were
available to lower the blood pressure and it had been well established that blood pressure elevations presented a definite
health risk. It was not until the late 1960's, however, that
definitive evidence was available that lowering blood pressure
made a difference, that it did indeed reduce the person's risk.
Using another popular example, cholesterol, we currently have
drugs which will lower the level of cholesterol in blood. We
also know that modifying the diet can result in reduced levels
of serum cholesterol. We know that cholesterol elevations are
associated with increased risk of cardiovascular disease. The
rub arises in that there is, to date, virtually no evidence
which demonstrates that lowering serum cholesterol levels also
lowers the risk of cardiovascular disease. Until such evidence
is available, it is of questionable value to market cholesterol
lowering as an available option.

The role of marketing in terms of raising awareness of
available options is clear. A long cited social redeeming factor of advertising is the service it provides in making consumers aware of the options available to them. In this writer's
opinion, there are few limitations on this marketing activity
other than availability of resources to circulate the information and the availability of channels through which to circulate
the information.

Figure 1

ADAPTATION OF THE HEALTH BELIEF MODEL *

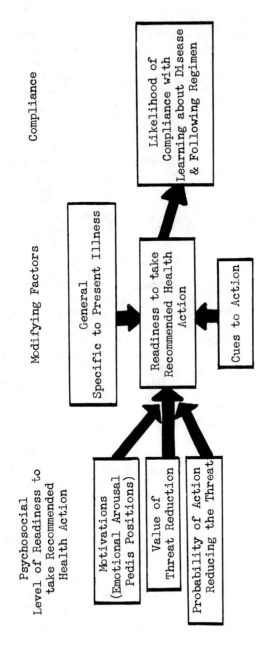

Psychosocial
Level of Readiness to
take Recommended
Health Action

Modifying Factors

Compliance

Motivations
(Emotional Arousal
Pedis Positions)

Value of
Threat Reduction

Probability of Action
Reducing the Threat

General
Specific to Present Illness

Readiness to take
Recommended Health
Action

Cues to Action

Likelihood of
Compliance with
Learning about Disease
& Following Regimen

*Adaptation & Health Belief Model as formulated by Marshall Becker
to predict compliance in pediatric study

75

Secondly, the necessity for the individual to understand the action in his own terms is essential. Using high blood pressure as an example, it is neither unreasonable nor atypical for a patient to ask, "I feel fine. Why should I take a pill every day, which I have trouble remembering to do, which costs me money and inconvenience to acquire it, and which makes me feel worse than I did before I learned I was supposed to be sick?" Even if the patient can say taking the pills will prevent a stroke or heart attack, that response may simply be parroting back words the provider has told him. If the patient can say taking the pills will help me live long enough to see my son graduate from college and to see my daughter bear children, this kind of understanding gets interest.

Marketing can contribute to achieving understanding but its limitation is inability of most marketing approaches to be specific to the individual. Since marketing efforts must use generalized examples which are designed to reach the largest possible segment of the audience, multiple messages and channels are required. The most severe limitation is securing adequate resources to produce the necessary messages for differing personalities.

The third critical point relates to the individual's capability of performing the action. A wide number of barriers may have to be overcome: physical, social, or economic. Recommending a healthy balanced diet of fresh fruits and vegetables to an inner-city ghetto community may be valid in theory but is impractical because of the economic barriers. Using another mundane example, tooth brushing, most of us would be astonished to learn how many people have never been specifically taught the necessary skills to effectively clean their teeth. Or what about the skills necessary for a lay person to extract personally usable information from a highly trained and technically oriented health professional. Consumers and patients require not only information but skill-learning. In the High Blood Pressure Education Program three years' work were needed to define the skills and attitudes which must be possessed by physicians, nurses and pharmacists to achieve high blood pressure control. However, the same analysis from the patient's point of view was not conducted, but we are now attempting to remedy that deficiency. The limitations in marketing these skills arise primarily from the fact that any given medium can effectively transmit only a limited amount of instruction in a given message unit. The implication is that we must develop a wide variety of messages and plan their delivery in an orderly and understandable sequence over an extended period of time.

CONCLUSION

In terms of marketing preventive health measures, we must also recognize our own capability limitations. It has been widely published that the three major killers in our Nation are heart disease, cancer and stroke. Exception can be taken to that statement. An alternative proposal would be: the major killers in our country are poverty, ignorance and apathy. It is within the role and capability of marketing to address ignorance and apathy. We exceed our bounds in attempting to resolve all the problems arising from poverty.

The final point deals with the payoff for certain actions and their perceived values. As mentioned earlier, it is our responsibility to ascertain what and whether a given action has a payoff. The state-of-the-art of preventive medicine must be such that we can define a cause and effect of a given action. In terms of marketing, we must not only possess this information, but we must also be able to ascertain some of the likely competing actions and their payoffs.

As a closing statement, preventive health care marketing is clearly limited by the potential of preventive health care. Once again, let us take hypertension as an example. In Table 1a are probabilities for success in achieving the four steps of hypertension control: detection, referral, selection of correct therapy and a two-year maintenance of control. Table 1a describes the probabilities in a typical community program. The overall net yield is approximately 10 Percent effectiveness as indicated in the final number of the right hand column.

In Table 1b two alternative approaches are presented, both of which achieve a final result of 20 Percent effectiveness. This table indicates that emphasis on varying steps can produce the same outcome. However, the likelihood of success in achieving a 100 Percent effectiveness in detection is very remote, but it is possible to increase the frequency with which correct therapy is selected and to increase the number of people who are maintained under control for a significant period.

Table 1c directly addresses the limitations of the system. It assumes that each event occurs at a very high effectiveness level, 85 Percent. When multiplied together, the net result is an overall effectiveness of 52 Percent. Thus, the overall success of any preventive medicine process which requires a series of events is limited by the cumulative, multiplicative success of each event and its subsequent events.

HIGH BLOOD PRESSURE CONTROL PROCESS
TYPICAL PROBABILITIES

	p^{Event}	$p^{Overall}$
Detection	.50	.50
Referral	.50	.25
Correct Therapy	.80	.20
Maintain Control (2 years)	.50	.10

Table 1b - ALTERNATIVE PROBABILITIES

	p^{Event}	$p^{Overall}$	*	p^{Event}	$p^{Overall}$
Detection	.50	.50	*	1.00	1.00
Referral	.50	.25	*	.50	.50
Correct Therapy	.90	.23	*	.80	.40
Maintain Control (2 years)	.85	.20	*	.50	.20
			*		
			*		

Table 1c - ALTERNATIVE PROBABILITIES

	p^{Event}	$p^{Overall}$
Detection	.85	.85
Referral	.85	.72
Correct Therapy	.85	.61
Maintain Control (2 years)	.85	.52

Regardless of the investment and the associated marketing effort, the hope of achieving 100 Percent success in this type of endeavor is assumed to be fruitless and frustrating. One marketing action which must occur is clear and rational representation of the success possibilities. On many occasions an unnecessary limitation arises through the marketing process, the projection of unfulfillable expectation. This pitfall must be scrupulously avoided.

REFERENCE

1. Baily, Richard M. Inquiry, 6:1 (1969).

IV. B. FROM THE ACADEMIC VIEW

The viewpoints of academics on problems and limitations of preventive health care and marketing are encapsulated here in papers by Dale D. Achabal, Robert J. Eng, Mark Moriarty and Reed L. Morton.

MARKETING AND PREVENTIVE HEALTH CARE: THE HMO EXAMPLE

Dale D. Achabal

BACKGROUND

Preventive health care delivery in the United States has experienced significant growth over the past decade. The prototypes of these prepaid health plans, or Health Maintenance Organizations (HMOs), are generally considered to be those developed on the West Coast by Kaiser Permanente and in the East by the Health Insurance Plan (HIP) of New York [10]. While the Kaiser and HIP plans have been successful, their impact on improving the delivery of health care in the U.S. has been less than overwhelming. However, HMOs present a viable and often preferred method of delivery over the existing system, or a reformed system based on nationalized health insurance or public ownership and management of health organizations.

A significant impetus to the development of HMOs was provided by Congress through the passage of the Health Maintenance Organization Act of 1973 (P.L. 93-222) which provided $375 million to encourage the planning and development of HMOs as a viable alternative to the dominant fee-for-service system [3]. This legislation has stimulated the formation of a number of profit and nonprofit HMOs across the U.S.   Rothfeld [13] and others view this very positively and estimate the development of $12.5 billion industry within the $150 billion health market projected for the mid-1980's.

The potential contribution of marketing to this growth has been evidenced in the publication of several studies discussing the need for marketing in the planning, development, and long-run success of HMOs [1,2,14,15]. However the imminent impact of HMO marketing is not seen to be very pervasive in the future for two basic reasons. First, a conceptual/philosophical issue exists with respect to the interpretation of marketing concepts in these past studies. There has been, without exception, a tendency to equate marketing and selling. Second, the perception of an HMO vis a vis the existing system varies significantly among the multi-publics which are either directly or indirectly

79

involved in the delivery or use of preventive health care. This complexity makes the incorporation of an integrated marketing strategy extremely difficult when compared to the traditional profit-oriented arena of marketing.

CONCEPTUAL ISSUES

Traditionally, marketing has been restricted to the profit oriented sector of our economy. Those involved in nonprofit organization have in recent years had a tendency to equate marketing and selling. This should not be taken as a criticism limited solely to nonprofit organizations. Levitt's [9] classic article dealing with the myopic view of profit oriented firms also dealt directly with this issue. He pointed out that, "The difference between marketing and selling is more than semantic. Selling focuses on the needs of the seller, marketing on the needs of the buyer." There are still a significant number of firms today that do not truly understand this distinction and its implications when formulating a marketing strategy.

The literature discussing HMO marketing is replete with studies that equate marketing and selling. A comprehensive study conducted by Texas Instruments, Inc. [14] deals directly with the establishment of marketing planning goals; however, the emphasis is placed on the specifics associated with generating sales from various groups rather than on the development of an integrated marketing plan. This study was followed by one conducted by Bionetics Research Laboratories [1] which emphasized the marketing of HMO services. This multi-volume publication detailed the methodology appropriate to segmenting the user population without discussing the formulation of an integrated plan to carryout an effective marketing program.

Two additional studies warrant brief discussion. The Department of Health, Education, and Welfare [15] sponsored a collection of papers that also equated marketing and selling. Probably the 'best' example to be taken from this volume is a list of 'good marketing practices' developed by Lanigan [8] -- be aggressive, be honest, meet a need, sell, get the check, run like hell, ..., always treat a customer like a prospect. Further, a study conducted by Burke [2] also ostensibly deals with HMO marketing, but the reader is referred to the TI, Bionetics, and HEW publications for work done on the more general problems of marketing (selling) HMOs.

MULTI-PUBLIC PERCEPTIONS

Kotler and Zaltman [7] define social marketing as the "design, implementation, and control of programs calculated to influence the acceptability of social ideas and involving consi-

derations of product planning, pricing, communication, distribution, and marketing research." Further, the authors note that,
"Too often social advertising rather than social marketing is
practiced by social campaigners." One of the most integral
facets of social marketing is the concept of a public. A public is a distinct group of people and/or organizations that have
an actual or a potential interest and/or impact on an organization [6]. An HMO interfaces with at least five different publics and must attain the support of each (1) users, (2) physicians, (3) hospitals, (4) intermediaries (e.g., Blue Cross/Blue
Shield), and (5) financial entities (e.g., foundations and/or
government).

What we have seen as a stimulus to the past growth of HMOs
is a small portion of each of the above publics who have readily
adopted the prepaid form of health care delivery. In innovation
diffusion terminology, these first adopters may be considered
innovators -- those who readily accept a new concept because it
more readily meets their needs. Unfortunately these individuals
do not tend to be the opinion leaders of their respective publics and are viewed as being 'venturesome' and willing to take
risks [12]. Further, what is of critical importance is how the
members of each of the publics perceive the relative innovativeness of the HMO concept.

Robertson [11] has formulated a classification system based
on the impact the innovation has on the social system accepting
the innovation. He classified a "continuous innovation" as one
which has the least disrupting influence on established behavioral patterns. Finally, a "discontinuous innovation" would
represent a truly new concept which would result in the formation of totally new behavioral patterns. This taxonomy is extremely relevant with respect to the complex multi-public interaction with HMOs as the relative innovativeness of the concept
varies across publics, as well as, segments within publics.
Herein lies the difficulty of the marketing task.

A brief analysis of three of the relevant publics will suffice to illustrate the complexity of the situation (see Figure
1). For physicians, the HMO might be viewed as a discontinuous
innovation since it will require the formation of new behavioral
patterns with respect to both the delivery of health care, as
well as, their method of remuneration. In an HMO the emphasis
is placed on preventive care rather than curative medicine and
is typically provided in a group practice environment. Further,
doctors would no longer be compensated under a fee-for-service
system, but rather would receive remuneration via prepaid capi-
tation payments. It is evident why the HMO concept has received
such vocal opposition from many professional medical societies.

Figure 1

POSSIBLE CLASSIFICATION OF HMO'S
AS INNOVATIONS ACROSS PUBLICS

| | Innovation Classification | | |
Public	Continuous	Dynamically Continuous	Discontinuous
Users		X	
Physicians			X
Hospitals		X	
Intermediaries	X		
Financial Entities	X		

A second view would be held by the users/subscribers to the system. An HMO may be viewed as a dynamically continuous innovation by many users as the concept stresses the preventive aspects of health care -- not necessarily conceptually different in the users mind, but operationally incongruous with the dominant existing health care delivery system in the United States.

A third public, the intermediaries, would continue to be involved as third parties in most situations and may view the HMO concept as a continuous innovation. Burke [2] has recommended the use of such intermediaries as 'third-party' representatives to sell the HMO to selected segments of the user/subscriber public under a contractual arrangement. This alternative has been utilized successfully by many of the existing HMOs. In this situation the intermediaries continue to be involved in providing a form of prepaid health insurance to individuals and groups with a minimum of disruption of their existing method of operation.

While the above categorization is clearly open to discussion, the salient point is the perceptual differences which exist in the eyes of alternative publics. Further, given these differences, the adoption rate of HMOs would also be expected to vary across publics. The adoption rate is related to the perceived newness and salient attributes of the innovation. If an idea were seen as a continuous innovation, it would be adopted more rapidly than one perceived to be a discontinuous innovation. The impact of this on the complexity of the marketing plan is evident of the possible classification schema presented in Figure 1 and is related to the adoption process.

Rogers and Shoemaker [12] have identified standardized adopter categories and distributions. The cumulative adopter distribution can be approximated by a S-shaped curve which is also of the same shape as the traditional product life cycle curve used in marketing. The product life cycle concept identifies the interrelationships between a product's (service) stage in the life cycle and marketing strategy. To be maximally effective each of the elements of the marketing mix -- service, distribution, price, and promotion -- should be coordinated to the appropriate stages of the product life cycle (adoption process). This situation would lead to an extremely complex strategy since an integrated marketing program would have to explicitly consider these factors.

CONCLUSION

These problems are clearly not insurmountable. The fact that this workshop has been organized attests to the potential cooperation and collaboration that will hopefully resolve some of these issues. What is more critical, however, is the complexity of marketing task which faces all of us once we move beyond the relatively superficial level of HMO marketing that has prevailed in the past. If we are to develop the HMO as a truly viable form of health care delivery in the future, we must understand clearly the potential that social marketing has to contribute to this industry.

REFERENCES

1. Bionetics Research Laboratories, Inc. Health Maintenance Organization Services Technical Assistance Publication. Marketing of Health Maintenance Organization Services. Washington, D.C.: Government Printing Office, 1972.

2. Burke, Richard T. Guidelines for HMO Marketing. Minneapolis: InterStudy, 1973.

3. Dorsey, Joseph L. "The Health Maintenance Organization Act of 1973 (P.L. 93-222) and Prepaid Group Practice Plans." Medical Care 8 (January, 1975), 1-9.

4. Kotelchuck, David (ed.). Prognosis Negative. New York: Vintage Books, 1976.

5. Kotler, Philip. "A Generic Concept of Marketing." _Journal of Marketing_ 36 (April, 1972), 46-54.

6. Kotler, Philip. _Marketing for Nonprofit Organizations_. Englewood Cliffs, New Jersey: Prentice-Hall, Inc. 1975.

7. Kotler, Philip, and Zaltman, Gerald. "Social Marketing: An Approach to Planned Social Change." _Journal of Marketing_ 35 (July, 1971), 3-12.

8. Lanigan, John. "The Marketing of a Prepaid Group Practice." In the U.S. Department of Health, Education and Welfare. _Marketing Pre-paid Health Care Plans_. Rockville, Maryland: Health Services and Mental Health Administration, Community Health Service/Health Maintenance Organization Service, July, 1972, pp. 18-26.

9. Levitt, Theodore. "Marketing Myopia." _Harvard Business Review_ 38 (July-August, 1960), 45-46.

10. Mechanic, David. _Public Expectations and Health Care_. New York: Wiley-Interscience, 1972.

11. Robertson, Thomas S. "The Process of Innovation and the Diffusion of Innovation." _Journal of Marketing_ 31 (January, 1967), 14-19.

12. Rogers, Everett M., and Shoemaker, F. Floyd. _Communication of Innovations_. New York: The Free Press, 1971.

13. Rothfeld, Michael B. "Sensible Surgery for Swelling Medical Costs." _Fortune_ (April, 1973).

14. Texas Instruments, Inc. Health Maintenance Organization Service Technical Assistance Publication. _The Development of an Implementation Plan for the Establishment of a Health Maintenance Organization_. Washington, D.C.: Government Printing Office, 1971.

15. U.S. Department of Health, Education and Welfare. _Marketing Pre-paid Health Care Plans_. Rockville, Maryland: Health Services and Mental Health Administration, Community Health Service/Health Maintenance Organization Service, July, 1972.

PREVENTIVE HEALTH CARE AND MARKETING:
SOME MISCONCEPTIONS

Robert J. Eng

The purpose of this paper is to put forth a single marketer's perceptions of some impediments to the development of an effective and efficient working relationship between marketers and preventive health care (PHC) planners, a relationship which if developed properly, could result in PHC as routinized behavior among the public. More specifically, this paper focuses upon 1) the problems due to a) misconceptions of the nature of marketing activities by PHC planners and b) misconceptions by marketers of what can be done for PHC, and 2) the constraints or limitations imposed upon the working relationship between marketers and PHC planners.

IMPEDIMENTS TO DEVELOPMENT OF
A WORKING RELATIONSHIP BETWEEN
MARKETERS AND PHC PLANNERS

PHC PLANNERS' MISCONCEPTIONS OF THE SCOPE OF MARKETING ACTIVITIES

Galiher and Costa, in a study of consumer acceptance of Health Maintenance Organizations (HMO) across the country, wrote a statement which perhaps exemplifies common view of the marketing function held by many PHC planners:

The staffs of most of the (HMO) plans that we visited expressed a need for guides - guides that spelled out precisely how to educate consumers, win consumer understanding and enroll consumers. [2, p. 106]

Marketing is perceived by many PHC staffers as simply an enrollment activity, a selling activity that takes place after organization plans have been finalized. For example, in most HMOs throughout the country, the marketing department is simply a group of persons charged with the responsibility of enrolling eligible consumers.

This narrow perspective of marketing has resulted (and will continue to result in the future) in lost opportunities for PHC planners. A major assumption by many PHC planners has been that any health program that gives benefits (from the eyes of the planners) will naturally attract consumers. Unfortunately, in the situation where consumer participation in such programs is voluntary, and the danger of illness is not perceived as immediate, consumer acceptance cannot be assured even with active

85

solicitation of enrollment. In the case of HMOs, enrollments have generally been below expectations [2, p. 106] and in one particular plan the enrollment rates have been only 5% to 20% of eligible consumers [8, p. 1].

The proper perspective of marketing should be:

Marketing is the analysis, planning, implementation and control of carefully formulated programs designed to bring about voluntary exchanges of values with target markets for the purpose of achieving organizational objectives. It relies heavily on designing the organization's offering in terms of the target markets' needs and desires, and on using effective pricing, communication and distribution to inform motivate and service the markets. [5, p. 5]

With this expanded view, it is possible for marketing to contribute to such decisions as market identification, formulation of product concept, pricing, distribution and promotion. Proper selection of target markets will increase the changes of efficient enrollment activity. In an assessment of the poor performance of the Columbia (Maryland) Medical Plan, Heyssel and Seidel [3, p. 1228] suggested that plans similar to Columbia Medical require selection of sizable population bases in order to increase the likelihood of financial viability. Perhaps selection of markets should be based upon factors other than just size of population or demographics; perhaps selection of markets at points in time should be based upon the psychological readiness to accept PHC as reflected in attitudes and lifestyles which may be identified by marketers.

With respect to product concept, it should be remembered that a desirable product in the eyes of the designer (in this case, the PHC provider) is not necessarily a desirable product in the eyes of the consumer. Many PHC planners tend to forget that preventive health care is considered discretionary by many of today's consumers. Unless the consumers themselves clearly see PHC as fulfilling a void in their medical needs, they will not give up their present health care habits. Marketing research is able to supply information concerning consumers' perceptions.

If a PHC program is dependent upon revenue directly from the consumers for financial viability, then marketing may be able to contribute with respect to pricing strategy. Price should not be viewed solely in the context of covering costs; depending on the target market, price should be viewed as a potential benefit or detriment to the overall product image. Marketing can provide proper guidance in pricing.

86

With respect to distribution, a factor very frequently cited by persons who elected to not subscribe to HMOs has been the inconvenience of the location. Planners of comprehensive PHC programs should consider the long term implications of location decisions as opposed to the short term benefits of housing all services under one roof or the convenience of existing facilities. PHC providers should avail themselves of techniques from marketers for the determination of optimum locations.

Promotion decisions are decisions concerning the communication of ideas. Many PHC providers have recognized the need for dissemination of information and marketers are in a position to provide expertise concerning what to say, in what vehicle to say it and how to say it. Of all marketing variables, this is perhaps the most recognized and accepted function of marketing among PHC providers.

MARKETERS' MISCONCEPTIONS OF THE OPPORTUNITIES IN PHC

One problem which has limited marketers is the stereotyping of their skills as being limited to the generation of profits through sale of items such as deodorants and toothpaste. Several marketers have attempted to have their concepts of marketing. In 1968, Robert Bartels [1] conceptualized marketing as an activity undertaken by society at large to meet its consumption needs for human existance; activity for economic gain is merely one aspect of marketing. In 1969, Kotler and Levy [6] called upon marketing people to expand their thinking and apply their skills to an increasingly interesting range of social activities; marketing people should not narrowly define marketing as a business activity. In 1971, Kotler and Zaltman [7] formally proposed the concept of social marketing which was defined as "the design, implementation and control of programs calculated to influence the acceptability of social ideas and involving considerations of product, planning, communication, distribution and marketing research." Presently, conferences such as this one may be encouraging indicators of broadened perspectives among marketers.

Another problem obstructing the development of an effective and efficient working relationship between marketers and PHC planners has been a reluctance on the part of marketers to actively seek out PHC opportunities due to beliefs that PHC providers would not be receptive to marketers' advances. That is, in the past, PHC providers have had the tendency to view marketing as simply the "hard-sell" and thus they would not be responsive to any suggestions to fully utilize marketers' skills. Hopefully, with the not-too-successful experiences of early PHC programs, PHC providers may be more understanding of what marketing is and in turn the marketers lose whatever reluctance they may have in becoming involved with PHC.

SOME LIMITATIONS UPON THE WORKING RELATIONSHIP

POLITICAL ISSUES

The political issues stems from medical professional associations, congressmen and various lobbying groups. PHC and
marketers will find that professional associations such as the
American Medical Association may provide formidable opposition
to new and relatively radical (although better) health care
programs. This would mean that marketing efforts may very well
have to be employed far in advance of finalization of program
plans in order to win the blessings of influential organizations
such as the AMA. Congressmen may provide interference in that
they have duties to represent the interests of their constituencies and that these constituencies are likely to not have similar views on the planning and execution of PHC programs. As
in the case of any significant public issue, lobbying groups
will be present to voice their sentiments; it is probably an
understatement that these various lobbying groups will offer
opinions and recommendations which may be extremely heterogeneous.

LEGAL ISSUES

Legal factors may very well dampen the enthusiasm among
marketers and PHC providers. One example of previous legal
difficulties in the planning and execution of a comprehensive
PHC program has been the situation of HMOs where federal legis-
lation was needed to override some state laws prohibiting prepaid medical practice and/or practice of medicine by corporations [4, p. 756]. The point here is that a significant activity in the mutual working relationship between PHC providers
and marketers may very well be campaigning for legislative incentives and/or protection.

ETHICAL ISSUES

Finally, there is the ethical issue concerning the cooperation of marketers and PHC providers. Medicine is a profession
where marketing is viewed as client solicitation and the "hard-
sell." A major task for the proponents of PHC is to impress upon the medical profession that the planning and execution of
marketing activities in health care need not take the form of a
marketing program for deodorant. The objective of marketing is
the effective and efficient delivery of goods and/or services;
the means for achieving the objective need not be unethical.

CONCLUSION

In order for successful interaction between marketers and PHC planners to occur, each group must recognize all the opportunities and/or skills available from the other group. A limited perspective of the other's potential leads to inefficient utilization of resources and thus suboptimization of performance.

The working relationship between marketers and PHC providers may have to devote a significant amount of effort to hurdling political, legal and ethical issues.

REFERENCES

1. Bartels, Robert, "The General Theory of Marketing", Journal of Marketing, January, 1968, pp. 29-33.

2. Galiher, Claudia and Marjorie Costa, "Consumer Acceptance of HMOs", Public Health Reports, March-April 1975, pp. 106-112.

3. Heyssel, Robert and Henry Seidel, "The Johns Hopkin Experience in Columbia, Maryland", The New England Journal Of Medicine, Vol. 295, No. 22 (11/25/76), pp. 1225-1231.

4. "HMOs: Are They the Answer to Your Medical Needs?", Consumer Reports, October 1974, pp. 756-762.

5. Kotler, Philip, Marketing for Non-Profit Organizations, Englewood Cliffs, New Jersey: Prentice Hall, 1975.

6. _____, and Sidney Levy, "Broadening the Concept of Marketing", Journal of Marketing, January 1969, pp. 10-15.

7. _____, and Gerald Zaltman, "Social Marketing - An Approach to Planned Social Change", Journal of Marketing, July 1971, pp. 3-12.

8. Lubin, Joann S., "Prepaid Medical Plans Run Into Difficulties as Enrollment Falters", The Wall Street Journal, 2/11/75, pp. 1+.

PROBLEMS AND LIMITATIONS OF THE IMPLEMENTATION AND
DIFFUSION OF MARKETING PRACTICES IN PREVENTIVE CARE

Mark Moriarty

The primary concern of the medical practitioner has evolved
from preventing and treating acute diseases to combatting the
ill effects of chronic diseases [2]. It might logically be expected that a shift in concern from acute diseases to chronic
diseases would entail a different approach to delivering and
practicing health care. However, in the United States, the personnel, equipment, and facilities of the contemporary medical
system seem to be established according to the classic or acute
care form of delivery [2]. Telling evidence of the imbalance in
national health care expenditures is noted for a recent year,
1972. In that year, 92% of the $95 billion spent for medical,
hospital or health care was expanded for treatment after illness
had occurred. More than half of the remainder was spent for
biomedical research. The remaining 3% was devoted to prevention of illness and consumer health education and promotion [7].

These data are suggestive of emphasis on detection subsequent to the onset of disease. Prevention and early detection
are not prominent in the existing domain of the health care system. In fact, preventive health care could be conceived as being an innovation with as yet a very low dollar share of the
health care market. A particular form or model of preventive
health care, the health maintenance organization (HMO) still has
attracted only a small share of eligible subscriber populations
[9].

It will be the contention of this paper that marketing
thought and practice can be utilized to promote the concept and
practice of preventive health care. Given this premise, the
purpose of the paper is to explore the problems and limitations
of using marketing to foster the diffusion of preventive health
care practices. Problems and limitations of particular interest
are those related to implementing preventive health care marketing strategies.

PROBLEMS

PRODUCT DELINEATION

Individual adoption of the concept of preventive health
care is quite meaningless unless reference is given to the context in which preventive actions are to be taken. Preventive
actions differ radically. Some require daily repitition, others

90

require sporadic action and still others are a one time action. They also vary in terms of the time, cost and discomfort required of the consumer. In a study by Williams [11], the issue of multiple preventive behaviors was studied. He found that six behaviors which relate to heart disease; namely, (1) medical checkups, (2) smoking, (3) exercise, (4) obesity, (5) limiting calories, and (6) cholesterol control, were not intercorrelated in terms of positive preventive action taken by respondents. Preventive health care advocates typically embrace the notion of multiple causation of chronic diseases. This should logically lead to promotion of not single actions but multiples of preventive actions which cumulatively reduce the risk of disease. It is not clear at this time that organizations which develop public programs seeking to influence people to take a preventive orientation recognize the need to have these programs be multifaceted to be maximally effective. That is, if the "product" is prevention of heart attack, the components of that product including all obvious preventive actions should be jointly promoted. Consumers need classifications of preventive actions (the total product) that relate to risk reduction for given diseases which are chronic in nature. When these are clearly defined, marketing has the technologies available to promote the product to appropriate populations.

MARKET DELINEATION

A difficulty with preventive health care is that there is not a dramatic change in immediate health status as a result of behaving preventively. Since the rewards of preventive behavior are deferred, it is likely that a consumer's time orientation has a significant impact on his/her predispositions with regard to adopting preventive health behaviors. Preventive health behavior is particularly congruent with sub-groups in society which have a predominantly future orientation [8]. Regarding health behavior, lower social classes, which do not display a future orientation, have been found not to believe in the asymptomatic presence of disease [5]. In somewhat the same vein, various socio-economic classes have been found to differ significantly in terms of their knowledge, attitudes, and behavior toward preventive health measures [1,4,10].

These studies strongly suggest that unrealistic expectations may attend efforts to promote preventive health care. In marketing terms, the "market" for preventive health care is segmented. It is segmented in terms of predispositions to behave preventively, and these predispositions may be strongly rooted in cultural, social class, and ethnic norms which are highly resistant to change. Those sub-groups (market segments) which are disposed to behave preventively will respond to promotional efforts. The marketing problem is to define the market segments

91

with predispositions consistent with preventive health care in terms of their demographic and life style patterns. Once this task has been performed, promotional strategies to reach these markets can be developed using conventional marketing technologies.

THE PHYSICIAN AS THE DISTRIBUTOR OF HEALTH CARE

Prior experiences of consumer patients involving the patient-physician relationship are likely to play a major role in determining current health behaviors. Gillum and Barsky examined the nature of the physician-patient realtionship in terms of its impact on compliance. Among their findings, they report that: (1) good rapport and free communication between the physician and patient fostered compliance to medical recommendations, and (2) the communication to the patient should be clear so that the patient understands the recommended regimen and implements it [6]. Clearly, then, compliance and communication with the physician are positively related.

It seems clear, in addition, that the physician's preventive orientation will subsequently affect the patients' compliance with preventive regimens. Such an orientation seems logically to be an extension and an outcome of physician training. Since medical schools supply doctors, the prevailing medical philosophy and orientation of the nation's medical schools seems to be the source of the preventive vs. the acute care orientation. If medical schools change or adopt a preventive orientation, it is likely that the physician populations educated at such schools will become essentially change agents which will facilitate transference of a preventive orientation to patient consumers. Evidence from rural sociology suggests that an analogous process operates for the dissemination of agricultural innovations among farm populations.

The long-run marketing task then is to convince medical schools to change their organizational philosophy and policies to reflect a preventive orientation. Some success with this strategy has been evidenced in dentistry and other allied health fields such as nursing. A perhaps short-run goal is to identify in the present physician population those with a preventive orientation who are also opinion leaders among their peers. If this task can be accomplished, it may be possible to motivate them to successfully "market" their orientation among their peers who represent the distributive agents of health care.

LIMITATIONS

With respect to product delineation, a central limitation will be the implementation of strategies which equally emphasize

92

the multiple preventive behaviors which should be engaged in to reduce the risk of later disease. A relatively new tool called health hazard appraisal, which has been developed for physicians practicing prospective medicine, shows promise for alleviating the problem of demonstrating multiple causality of chronic diseases to patients. It shows people's risks in perspective, demonstrates the quantitative and interactive nature of risk taking behaviors, and points out the personal relevance and immediacy of threats to their health [3].

In terms of market delineation, a critical limitation from the perspective of the health community will be the acceptance of a market segmentation approach. In all likelihood, a total market approach to promoting preventive health behaviors will be viewed as the ethical stance since it is the non-exclusionary alternative which does not view people's status differently.

The major limitation in relying on the physician to facilitate the transference of a preventive orientation to patients is revealed in an examination of the physicians' motives for adopting the acute model of health care delivery. Physicians typically see their key function as healing the sick and the injured, not describing preventive measures to patients which sometimes have an uncertain and deferred reward. There is also typically less financial reward for the physician who adopts the preventive model of health care.

REFERENCES

1. Coburn, David and Clyde R. Pope. "Socioeconomic Status and Preventive Health Behavior," Journal of Health and Social Behavior, 8 (June 1974), p. 67.

2. Coe, Rodney M. and Henry P. Brehm. Preventive Health Care for Adults (New Haven, College and University Press, 1972).

3. Colburn, H. N. and P. M. Baker. "Health Hazard Appraisal - A Possible Tool in Health Protection and Promotion," Canadian Journal of Public Health, 64 (September-October, 1973), p. 490.

4. Dennison, Darwin. "Social Class Variables Related to Health Instructions," American Journal of Public Health, 62 (June, 1972), p. 814.

5. Douglass, Chester W. "A Social-Psychological View of Health Behavior for Health Services Research," Health Services Report, 6 (Spring, 1971), p. 9.

6. Gillum, Richard F. and Arthur J. Barsky. "Diagnosis and Management of Patient Noncompliance," Journal of the American Medical Association, 228, (June 19, 1974), p. 1563-67.

7. Kennedy, Edward. National Disease Control and Consumer Health Education and Promotion Act of 1975 - - Report, 93rd Congress, 1st Session, 1466 (1975), p. 24.

8. Knutson, Andie L. The Individual, Society and Health Behavior, (New York: Russell Sage Foundation, 1965), p. 107.

9. Kotler, Philip. Marketing for Nonprofit Organizations, Englewood Cliffs, New Jersey: Prentice Hall, Inc., 1975, p. 315.

10. Shaw, Clay T. "Class Characteristics of Supporters and Rejectors of Basic Health Measures," Social Science and Medicine, 4 (November, 1970), pp. 411-5.

11. Williams, Allan F. and Henry Wechsler. "Interrelationship of Preventive Actions in Health and Other Areas," Health Service Report, 87, (December, 1972), pp. 969-76.

PROBLEMS IN HOSPITAL MARKETING OF PREVENTIVE HEALTH SERVICES

Reed L. Morton

The concern of this paper is the set of problems anticipated in marketing preventive health services through a hospital. Immediately issues of definition arise, especially in regard to the concepts of hospital, marketing and preventive health care services. As this paper is intended to stimulate discussion, it also seems essential to consider the assumption hospitals are an appropriate agency to involve in preventive health service marketing.

THE CONCEPT OF HOSPITAL

Hospitals are social institutions with a long history. As with other structures institutionalized to meet a recurring need of societies, over their history hospitals have received different assignments from their predominating cultures. Caring-- for travelers, for poor, and afflicted--was the initial responsibility. More recently, curing has predominated. As technical

94

workshop for physicians, and physician to large segments of a
mobile population, the hospital has evolved into the core of an
acute medical service delivery system.

Recently, recognition of the inevitable costlines of acute
treatment has drawn widespread concern to how hospitals consume
resources. Now, society is unwilling to assign resources and
responsibility for health care without more accountability and,
bluntly, more benefit for its monies. The result appears to be
a modification of the hospital's mission. It must move the
boundaries of care provided from medical to health care. It
must also measure the quantity of resources consumed, the quality of services provided, and the effectiveness of its entire
undertaking. If the hospital finally becomes an effective community health resource, it is foreseeable the information func-
tion--serving physician and regulator needs--could rival caring
for primacy.

THE CONCEPT OF MARKETING

The second definition concerns the concept of marketing
which may be considered the formalized logic of distribution.
However, if it is to enjoy the dignity of such a title, marketing probably must forego any claims to a twenty century history.
Actually, a twentieth century history has been sufficient to
include a break first from the "dismal science", economics, and
then, with Professor Kotler's impetus, a break from business.
For present purposes, however, a definition of marketing suggested by a voice on the narrower, business-only side of marketing seems appropos. Professor Robert Bartels of Ohio State University constructed the following definition to be consistent
with a general theory of marketing:

Marketing is the process whereby society, to supply
its consumption needs, evolves distributive systems
composed of participants, who, interacting under con-
straints--technical or ethical--create the transactions
which resolve market separations and result in exchange
and consumption.

To begin the transition to the health care sector requires only
substituting health care delivery for marketing, health care
needs for consumption, and provider-patient for market. To complete the transition involves considering the technical and
ethical constraints.

THE CONCEPT OF PREVENTIVE HEALTH CARE

The final concept to define is the product--preventive
health care. John van Steenwyk developed a useful hierarchial

95

model of preventive health services (<u>Blue Cross Reports</u>, 1969).
Primary prevention--most basic--includes immunization, infectious disease control and environmental sanitation. Secondary prevention involves periodic check-ups and early disease detection. Tertiary prevention requires early sickness consultation with a physician. Looking on secondary prevention as the weakest link in this chain, van Steenwyk suggested prevention could be obtained effectively with a system of prevention. Its components include:

- a broad range of physiological measures-multiphasic screening
- a physical exam by a physician
- appropriate health education materials
- facilities for referral

The hoped for outcomes are improved health levels in the population and greater return on the social investment in health care servcies.

MARKETING PREVENTIVE HEALTH SERVICES

With definitions in hand, the priority becomes examining the assumption hospitals should have the responsibility for marketing preventive health services. For discussion, a summary of major points pro and con should suffice. Advocates of the hospital as marketer have pointed out:

1. Hospitals have or should have concern with the entire spectrum of health.

2. A team approach is an essential ingredient to a preventive health system and the team already exists in the hospital organization.

3. Hospitals have necessary supportive facilities and resources, including a developing evaluative orientation and capacity.

4. Hospitals already serve as physician equivalents for many in the population.

Opponents offer a number of reservations:

1. This is another area for potentially expensive and wasteful duplication of services.

2. Physician preeminence would tend to exclude community input and stifle participation.

3. Hospitals would reach those already sick to the exclusion of those not already patients.

4. Hospitals cannot afford to monitor compliance and effectiveness.

Ultimately, the issue may turn on the incentives given the hospital by the many publics with which it exchanges influence. For now, granting hospitals the marketer role will permit consideration of how present incentives and the technical and ethical constraints mentioned earlier impinge on hospital management of the marketing mix.

Marketing management can be considered a managerial philosophy embodying a democratic technology. Cast as a technology, its reliance on tools is clear. The tools are familiar as the marketing mix, the four P's: product, price, promotion, and place. Application requires adding the fifth and silent "P" -- marketing research. It is this last element which, when effectively conducted, gives marketing its democratic character. Knowledge produced by research informs providers of consumer needs, attitudes and market behaviors. Decisions become based on votes measured in the marketplace.

MARKET RESEARCH

Placing a research function with a preventive health service marketing hospital seems indispensable; however, one ethical and one technical constraint looms large. Confidentiality of medical recods is virtually synonymous with the inviolable trust characterizing doctor-patient realtionships. The need to know--physiological, hereditary, life-style data--strikes at individual rights to privacy. Violating ethical expectations of physicians and patients risks alienating two publics vital to successful preventive care marketing.

Beyond ethics, is the technical constraint of measured cost. Not only is information not free, it is expensive. Hospitals cannot reasonably be expected to incur information costs without full economic reimbursement. Implicit in an exchange of hospital research for government or insurer dollars is recognizing value in research dictating "no go" on a program. Admittedly, hospitals may not yet have a record of saying no often enough, but incentives have not encouraged negative decisions.

PRODUCT

Product decisions face technical constraints. Thanks to van Steenwyk's model, the tangible product is specified as second stage preventive care--an early disease detection system.

97

Again, reimbursement for providing the service remains an issue.
The core product, long-run improvement of health status, presents promotional problems when considering consumers. Reim-
bursers, however, seek accountability in terms of quality assurance. Again, dollars and energy must be added to hospitals'
production function, implicitly trading initially higher hospital costs for presently intangible long-run gains. If resource
levels don't increase, the trade-off is less medical care for
those presently intangible benefits. A clear implication is a
diminished right to health for consumers seeking other services
in the ever-broadening hospital product line.

PRICE

Price setting presents few problems, although an active
Federal Trade Commission might find collusive elements in nego-
tiated reimbursement policies. It is on the consumer side that
issues arise. To date, demand for free preventive measures has
been quite elastic (Detroit recently barred from schools those
children unimmunized, despite free services at outreach centers).
Negative financial prices may be necessary. Non-financial costs
--time, energy--must be minimized to consummate exchanges with
consumers who, judging from life-styles, do not value preventive
measures.

PLACE

Place decisions raise alternatives dealing with marketing
agents, locations, and time of service delivery. Efficiency
dictates using non-physicians for any preventive service except
diagnosis and prescription. Among market segments accustomed
to dealing exclusively with doctors in health matters, the intrusion of less highly qualified medicos in their health process may be resisted. The regionalizing, rationalizing trends
in hospital service location present a technical problem. Efficiency concerns of providers may not result in service sites
convenient for consumers predisposed to avoid preventive services. Health planning agencies may be forced to permit duplication which otherwise would be abhorred. If assured of economic cost reimbursement, hospitals can be expected to compete in
offering these services.

PROMOTION

Promotion is the final concern. Ethical considerations
appear diminished in light of recent FTC actions against professional prohibitions on advertising. Consumer "ethics", however, are not subject to FTC rulings. The assumption that all
segments will appreciate hospital persuasion remains to be demonstrated. Hospitals' technical abilities to promote are ques-

tionable, too. This activity has been taboo and hospital administrators' experience is limited to annual reports, news releases and inducements to physicians to refer patients. Finally effective persuasion is costly. Again, this expense must be recognized in reimbursement.

CONCLUSION

In conclusion, the problems are many and the benefits questionable, long-term and intangible. Yet, this situation has prevailed for some time. Finally, the health strategy is apparent. Perhaps, at last, effective tactics will emerge. Hospital administration will respond to the proper incentives. It is hoped consumers will, too. Only through effective marketing will the answer emerge.

IV. C. FROM THE PRACTITIONER'S POINT OF VIEW

The pragmatic viewpoint of the practitioner as he/she perceives the problems and limitations of preventive health care and marketing is presented here in papers by Harold F. Pyke, William D. Novelli and James M. Summers.

INSURMOUNTABLE OPPORTUNITIES AND THE MARKETING OF PREVENTIVE HEALTH CARE

William D. Novelli

The assigned subject of this paper is perceived problems and limitations for marketing and preventive health care. Being a strong believer in the application of marketing techniques to health problem-solving, <u>opportunities</u>, rather than problems, will be discussed.

Perhaps, it is partly a question of semantics. A colleague, in a marketing corporation in New York, lived by the adage that there are no problems - only opportunities. This kind of logic brought him to eventually coin a phrase for delemmas that appeared to have no solutions. He called them, "insurmountable opportunities."

PROBLEMS

There are seven problems in marketing and preventive health care. Whether these seven issues represent problems or opportunities, and whether they are surmountable or not, depends on the thinking and action that results from workshops and conferences such as this one. The seven dilemmas are these:

99

1. The Difficulties of Measuring Results

We are not in the business of increasing retail distribution, or registering a gain in units sold or showing a bulge in
net profit. Our business is not without accountability, but the
bottom line is much more difficult to grab hold of. Goals are
broadly written and address such long-term needs as reductions
in morbidity and mortality. Objectives are often less global,
but equally difficult to measure. In the February, 1977 issue
of the American Journal of Public Health, Dr. Larry Green,
identified seven problems in measuring health education efforts.
He points out that methods of measurement common to other behavioral disciplines, including marketing, are not directly applicable to the problems of health.

Some of the projects in which we are now engaged include
smoking reduction and cessation, breast self examination, long-
term maintenance in anti-hypertensive drug therapy and prevention of drug addiction. Each of these areas represent difficult
measurement problems.

2. The Danger of a Fading Mandate

Today, a strong mandate exists. The National Consumer
Health Information and Health Promotion Act of 1976 calls for:

a.   The incorporation of appropriate health
     education components into our society, espe-
     cially into all aspects of education and
     health care.

b.   Increased incorporation of health knowledge,
     skills, and practices by the general popula-
     lation into its patterns of daily living.

c.   The establishment of systematic processes for
     the exploration, development, demonstration,
     and evaluation of innovative health promotion
     concepts.

And DHES's, Public Health Service, "Forward Plan For
Health", (For FY 1978-82, issued August 1976) outlines efforts
to assure that health education, health promotion, and preventive health services are emphasized in all Public Health Service
programs.

But, mandates and the dollars that go with them can be reduced, and diverted. What is needed are results. How does
money spent in prevention pay off? What approaches, strategies,
and health marketing mixes work best? To answer questions like

100

these, better measurement, which leads us backward, without "passing go," to the difficulties of evaluation is required.

3. Marketing as a Fad

In this writer's experience with the health community, current naughty words are "advertising," "slick," and "Madison Avenue." The concept of marketing, while not well understood, is currently accepted and in vogue. Health marketing is not a completely honest trade, mind you, but it appears to be generally acceptable. Dr. Philip Kotler, a prominent social marketer, believes that "each time marketing enters a new industry, it is opposed by the more conservative forces within that industry."

Two things are happening which treaten the continued acceptance of marketing in the field of health. First, the language of marketing is being used by individuals without full understanding of the underlying concepts. For instance, the use of the word "marketing" to mean "distribution," as in "now that we've got this poster produced, we've got to market it." Without a grasp and application of marketing concepts, the language of marketing will lose value and go out of vogue, as a vernacular whose time has come and gone.

Secondly, marketing professionals who know commercial marketing are attempting to apply their experiences directly to health. As one who has marketed laundry detergents, pet foods, toothpastes, and other household items, this writer believes that the techniques are transferrable, but not directly so. Health marketing is far more complex and difficult. Aside from the obvious differences in desired behavior outcomes, there are significant distinctions in such important areas as: primary and secondary target audience selection; strategy identification; motivation through consumer "benefits"; the weight and role of advertising as part of the overall marketing mix; utilization of a "sales" force and techniques and cost efficiencies in evaluation. If these differences are not understood, the application of commercial marketing techniques will be seen as misdirected and inappropriate by health professionals. When this happens, the concept of marketing in health may fall into disrepute.

4. Prevention Behavior - A Tough Sell

Clearly, prevention is essential to the improvement of public health. Much has been written about the difficulties of stimulating prevention behavior. For the purposes of outlining the problem suffice it to say that we are faced with motivating behavior change among individuals who perceive themselves to be healthy and who have little interest in our message. Part of this is the challenge of motivating lifestyle change. Is this,

101

perhaps, an insurmountable opportunity?

5. Lack of Training Opportunities

Most health programs, whether prevention programs or not, are managed at some level by the physician administrator. It has been said that physicians are trained for crisis management and not for prevention. However, the point is that physicians are most assuredly not grounded in marketing. Of course, this lack of familiarity with marketing approaches is not only true of physicians. Health planners and managers often gravitate to their positions from a broad variety of fields and academic disciplines. Few are trained in marketing or aware of its potential application to their programs.

In fact, there appears to be no training ground in social marketing per se. Actual, on-the-job experience must be gained in the commercial marketing sector, and then transferred, through trial and error, to the public sector.

6. Lack of Standardized Approaches and Norms

Larry Green's call for standardization in evaluation (noted above) applies to other aspects of health marketing as well. There is scant literature in social marketing applied to health. There is no handbook of techniques. A marketing corporations' library may contain hundreds of reports on, say, the use of product sampling as a technique in new product introductions. An advertising agency can review reams of television commercial recall data for a given product category. Granted, health education has its "literature", but since the application of marketing to health is relatively new, we have no compendium of health marketing results.

7. Shaping the Product or Service

In the marketing of commercial goods and services, the product must be shaped in response to consumer values and needs. If the product or service benefit is perceived by target consumers to be unimportant, unnecessary, personally irrelevant or for some other reason to be unappealing, the product is likely to fail in marketplace.

We often do not have the luxury of shaping our health prevention products or services. In many cases, we are hampered by lack of technology. In other instances, the product or service is shaped by the Congress and passed on to program managers. Thus, we may be in the position of offering a less than superior product to a consumer audience that feels healthy and is not predisposed to buy. As we all know, that is no way to corner a market.

102

CONCLUSION

There are other problems in health marketing, such as budget limitations, contracting red tape, lack of accountability and incentive, survey and other research delays and restrictions. But the seven problems briefly outlined above should be enough for workshop discussion.

Moreover, as stated earilier, this writer is a believer in health marketing and an optimist. While we don't have all the answers, and perhaps we are faced with many "insurmountable opportunities", the benefits of every success are great. The bottom line in our business is good health, lowered social costs, reductions in suffering, and the prolonging of human life.

PREVENTIVE HEALTH CARE MARKETING:
INNOVATIVE COMMUNICATION APPROACHES

Harold F. Pyke

Medical teaching and research centers and professional organizations have long been concerned with problems of continuing
medical education and have experimented with newer communications
technologies to help speed the flow of information from research
laboratories to practicing physicians. These efforts have
spawned a new field of specialization called biomedical communications. Still in its relative infancy, the field employs a variety of techniques to create substantive changes through education. Communications technology has been applied with varying
degrees of success to the following issues:

- Rising costs of health service.

- Rising expectations by consumers for better health care.

- Maldistribution of facilities and professional expertise.

- Difficulty of providing current continuing medical education, inservice training and access to modern facilities
  for isolated health practitioners.

- Tendency for medical school graduates to specialize.

- Difficulty of access to adequate health care in rural
  areas or inner-city slums.

PHYSICIAN EDUCATION

The emphasis has been on education of physicians, which can
be interpreted loosely as information dissemination or "lines of
communication." Other approaches to problem solving have been
pretty much ignored. Since the 1950's we have experimented with
intrafacility closed circuit television systems; public television networks; videotape distribution; interfacility closed circuit systems utilizing microwave and cable, both one-way and
two-way; and satellite communication. Most experiments were
initially funded through Federal grants. They died when money
ran out. After initial ripples of activity, most died without
leaving any noticeable changes in existing patterns of care. The
health care system has been virtually immune to education in the
classic sense; the institution is resistant to change.

104

CONSUMER HEALTH EDUCATION

The concept of consumer health education is also new to the health care system. As late as 1964, one state medical society refused to sanction use of public broadcast television for continuing medical education although assurances of propriety were offered. The reason given was that the public might accidently view a program and seek additional information on the subject from his physician. Times have changed somewhat. Now physicians and other health professionals seem to aggree that educating their patients to improve communication and cooperation is worthwhile. The public, in the race of rising costs, wants more information and believes that physicians and clinics are the best sources for it.

If there is general consensus, why hasn't there been systematic development of consumer education programs? Among the reasons offered are lack of financial incentive, there's no immediate, tangible benefit; marginal commitment by health professionals, "it's not our primary responsibility;" and lack of adequate research which links together information with improved patient care. Some of these issues are now being addressed by both public and private interests.

A July 1975 report of the Task Force on Consumer Health Education defined consumer health education as a set of activities which

#1. "Inform people about health, illness, disability and ways in which they can improve and protect their own health, including more efficient use of the delivery system;

#2. "Motivate people to want to change to more healthful practices;

#3. "Help them learn the necessary skills to adopt and maintain healthful practices and lifestyles;

#4. "Foster teaching and communications skills in all those engaged in educating consumers about health;

#5. "Advocate changes in the environment that facilitate healthful conditions and healthful behavior;

#6. "Add to knowledge via research and evaluation concerning the most effective ways of achieving the above objectives."

The report points out that any organization committed to

leadership in the field must be committed to the full range of activities. Clearly, narrowly based, piecemeal approaches to the problem will be inadequate.

Acceptance of consumer health education may be enhanced by actions resulting from a Blue Cross White Paper in which the association concludes that patient education can both increase the quality of care and present potential cost savings to the public it serves. Additional data are becoming available.

CONSUMER HEALTH EDUCATION EXAMPLES

A recent study conducted in five Indiana hospitals provides more substantive data upon which hospital administrators can begin to plan and implement effective patient education programs. Wells National Services Corporation (a subsidiary of American Hospital Supply Corp.) supplies hospitals with communications systems, so has an obvious interest in expanding the uses to which its patient systems can be put. In late 1974, it contracted with Throckmorton/Satin Associates, a N.Y. research and communications marketing firm, to explore the following issues:

1. To what extent would hospital patients watch health information programs on their television sets when they had regular TV fare to choose from as well?

2. For those patients who watched the programs, what, if any, information would be retained?

3. Did exposure to health education programs contribute to improved communications between patients and the nursing staff?

4. What were the most effective means of informing and motivating patients to view the programs?

The Medical Education Resources Program of Indiana University School of Medicine was asked to select and distribute programming to five large community hospitals in which MERP had ongoing professional educational programming through closed circuit television. Patients were provided program guides, reminder cards were distributed on lunch trays, and announcements were made to patients over hospital PA systems. Five different one-hour programs consisting of four or five short subject were televised twice each day. Hospitals appointed coordinators to help plan and implement the study and allowed patient demographic information to be given the researchers. Trained field survey teams conducted patient interviews each day following the telecasts. Substantial care was taken to involve medical professionals.

106

Wells National reported that use of master antenna connected TV sets in patients' rooms is an effective way of providing health information and education. Patients who viewed the programs (34.2%) indicated that they liked receiving the information on their TV sets and wanted to continue to see more programs of the type shown. The data showed that they could recall a significant number of important informational points after viewing a program. Nursing staff favored increased use of television for patient education (70.5%) and expressed need for additional education materials (79.1%). They also recommended use of supplementary materials to support the TV experience. The survey suggested that when patients are exposed to information in this way, nonpatients may be exposed as well.

OTHER EDUCATIONAL APPROACHES

Other innovative approaches to health information currently being explored include:

- Satellite communication: Various federal agencies and public organizations have begun an organized movement to use high powered satellites for public service communications. The recently formed Public Service Satellite Consortium is the focus of these efforts.

- MATV Systems (Master Antenna TV Systems): Suppliers of master antenna systems to hospitals, business, hotels, etc. are seeking new services to offer their customers and will need well produced programs to supply them.

- Broadband telemedicine networks: The WAMI project, Ohio Valley Medical Network and Dartmouth's Interact System have potential for consumer oriented health programming specifically tailored for regional needs. Initial trials have been moderately successful, but more development is required.

It appears, then that new information distribution channels may begin to make in roads on the health education market. But, issues of product design, point of entry and timing may be critical. Companies attempting to climb aboard the "knowledge explosion" bandwagon in the early to middle 60's by supplying education materials to the health industry were notably unsuccessful. A coordinated system for problem research, information dissemination and project action across several fronts is needed. The major reasons Federal programs fail at the local level are lack of adequate information and inability of local areas to organize to take advantage of the programs on a timely and effective basis.

CONCLUSION

We can capitalize on current experience to improve health education services capable of meeting a variety of demonstrated needs. Through efforts like the National High Blood Pressure Education Program, we are starting to acquire skills in dealing with professional organizations, disseminating information, helping state and local governments organize to cope with their problems, utilizing mass media and non-commercial media channels, and working closely and successfully across Federal agency boundaries. Additional skills can be combined into an efficient, functional system, we will be in position to develop with some assurance health information and education programs which depend upon broad based, local action for success.

PREVENTIVE HEALTH CARE: PERCEPTIONS OF RESPONSIBILITY

James M. Summers

Strolling into the mind's eye of the perceptive communica-
tor are wonders about the real knowledge that will pour from the
Cooper's, Kehoe's and Murphy's who have seen and pursued the
more direct causes for the conscious or unconscious problems in
health care. What this writer can offer to shade this research
in a positive direction is a sobering responsibility.

RESPONSIBILITY FOR PREVENTIVE HEALTH CARE

The transfer of the responsibility of preventive health
care to the individual is <u>almost</u> nonexistent. The structure
and systems of the body are covered with little attention given
to an educational program of maintenance for good, better, or
best health. Physical education is taught in many places with
the round or oblong ball with little emphasis on life-long exercise and diet. Food served at school or at home fail, for
many reasons, to satisfy preventive health needs.

Tradition and lack of knowledge defeat the ultimate goal
of optimal health. While the "Atomic Age" has brought diagnostic revolution, it did not bring with it the realization that
early prevention would be the better discovery. Education to
cope with change before it overtakes and affects our health is
now evident.

It is interesting to think about the great traditions of a
holiday meal in a farm kitchen, as compared with a modern holiday meal served at a restaurant. In a moment of thought about
the fresh products without the additives for color, taste, or
beauty is enough to wish for the H. G. Wells', <u>Time Machine</u>.
Traditions of food are being maintained in both quantity and
variety; however, the content is no longer consistent with good
health.

A second thought that goes with the great tradition of
foods, like mother made, is the next day or so afterward. Early
to rise, with a great day of physical activity to whittle away
the stored energy and to develop all manner of muscles, heart
and circulation to prevent a multitude of health problems.

Education has not overtaken traditions in sufficient depth
to change characteristic attitude and motivation toward better
individual health care. We eat too much of what we traditionally like, in quantities that are too large, with little exer-

cise to utilize its energy. We enjoy traditional good health and, therefore, concern is for health care at the surface level. Health care is for those with poor health.

Traditional diets with little realization that food content may be different; traditional quantities of food with little effort to use the energies it provides; TV and office occupations that help make us a technical nation, are traditionally adding to our need for preventive health care awareness. The conglomerate of traditions and the easy life are preventive health education barriers.

THE SCHOOL CURRICULUM

A second perception that may be of some value to question, is the lack of school curriculum emphasis. Several direct and related reasons for this lack of emphasis exist. The standard curriculum follows the pathways of how to get to college and how to learn a trade to support one's self. There seldom seems enough time to mix a priority such as preventive health, that seems not to affect the "now" of life. The questions of curriculum placement, adequate coverage, one-shot course vs. integrated within subjects, cost of programs and how to market it to motivate life-long learning and proper health patterns must be answered.

THE PHYSICIAN'S ROLE

The physician must be aware of the economic and financial aspects of private enterprise. Patient care may be paramount but it must generate income sufficient to insure financial safety. The "well patient" does little to add to the physician's income.

Medical schools teach the physician to diagnose and care for the sick patient. A majority of the supportive allied medical persons are trained to support maintenance and rehabilitation from the point of diagnosis through the well or ambulatory "normal" cycle. There seems to be no role, nor is there incentive, for the health professionals in preventive health care to provide education for the "well patient."

CONCLUSION

Preventive health care is an event waiting to happen. Marketing the experience is a systematic approach that will work. Health professionals are needed to disseminate information and the educational system seems the logical vehicle for delivery. Marketing is needed to create high public awareness levels and need for training. The more important factor may be to motivate a "life-long" program for individual preventive health care.

IV. D. PROBLEMS AND LIMITATIONS: SUMMARY COMMENTS

Summarizers' perceptions of the concurrent discussions of problems and limitations of preventive health care and marketing are included in this section. Included are comments of Ronald G. Blankenbaker, Angelo A. Alonzo and Lawrence H. Wortzel.

SUMMARY COMMENTS: PERCEPTIONS OF PROBLEMS AND LIMITATIONS OF PREVENTIVE HEALTH CARE AND MARKETING

Angelo A. Alonzo

Discussion focused on problems and limitations in merging marketing and preventive health care (PHC) from the perspectives of marketing, medicine, government and social policy. The following summarization highlights the discussion in terms of three issues or areas that were frequently addressed.

I. A primary issue of concern centered on whether marketing would be called upon to engage in product or social marketing. This issue was either manifestly or latently expressed in most every topic or comment raised. On the one hand, it was felt that marketing's general orientation and approach to problems is too short term to deal with intrinsic issues in PHC that relate to questions of life style or quality of life changes. In addition, it was pointed out that social marketing intended to change attitudes and values has not been very successful. Thus, there was a definite perceived need for a clear specification of PHC modalities that could be handled within a product marketing framework. What is needed is a product that can be shaped and delivered, quality of life issues were felt to be too abstract.

On the other hand it was argued that PHC is a much larger problem than a single deliverable modality such as a hypertension check. Further social change is, in fact, possible within short periods of time given that effective methods are used, for example, agricultural changes in underdeveloped countries have been quite successful. It was agreed that long-term changes in life style, if attempted by marketing would be incrementally small, but yet conceivably possible over the long run.

II. Various suggestions were made as to the type or point of PHC intervention. Each PHC modality appeared to be aligned with either a social or product marketing orientation. Intervention types are listed below, including some inducements and limitations to their application.

111

A. Physicians were initially seen as logical providers of
    PHC, albeit, at present, secondary rather than primary
    providers. However, physicians were not perceived as
    having enough time to educate patients, although it was
    felt that either economic inducements with the fee for
    service system or mandatory procedures within a nation-
    al health system could increase the delivery of primary
    PHC within the medical practice context. Also, changes
    in medical education and reorganization of the health
    care delivery system were touched upon.

B. The educational system was considered as an existing
    framework within which to socialize children toward PHC
    and healthful practices. Questions in this context were
    raised as to the most effective time and place to put
    PHC in the curriculum, and how PHC should be taught and
    by whom. Provisions for continuing education and the
    necessity of societal reinforcement of learned preven-
    tive practices was also stressed.

C. Though discussants tended toward a more persuasive than
    mandatory or legislative approach to encouraging PHC,
    there was consensus that much more could be done to al-
    ter the environment to bring about changes in the health
    status of individuals, for example, dietary changes at
    food manufacturing and processing points and improve-
    ments in occupational safety. The issue is to deter-
    mine when environmental change is the most efficient
    and effective means of promoting PHC.

D. At a somewhat abstract level, the discussion frequently
    turned to the issue of societal intervention to pro-
    mote PHC vs. small "cottage" type entrepreneurs of PHC
    modes. The governmental role was perceived as necessary
    for broad quality of life changes, but the prospect of
    a "Big Brother" image and a potential discontinuity of
    funding and priority were felt to be detriments to
    needed reinforcement and continuity of PHC activities.

        A "cottage" industry of individual entrepreneurs
    promoting specific PHC measures was at the other end of
    the continuum free of governmental intervention, albeit
    assisted in some way by federal funding. The federal
    government should make available resources for groups of
    physicians or nurse practitioners who wish to deliver
    PHC, and for other entrepreneurs who wish to promote
    inexpensive, convenient PHC modalities in shopping cen-
    ters, or wherever they are deemed to be effective on
    the basis of marketing studies.

E. At an even more abstract level, concern was expressed
    for the need for greater societal integration to over-
    come the segmental way in which health is divorced from
    other societal institutions and activities. If the
    marketing of PHC is going to be effective there needs to
    be integrated, persistent reinforcement from religion,
    the family and education. For example, there should be
    a greater concern in the schools for teaching sports
    that can be carried over to later life and even reli-
    gious institutions should promote PHC as having reli-
    gious significance; however, to convince the ministry
    of this later point may be beyond the scope of marketing.

III. Lastly, seven areas or topics were repeatedly referred to
     irrespective of what modality was selected or level of in-
     tervention proposed.

   A. Needs assessment is necessary to determine what consum-
       ers consider PHC and what they desire in the area of PHC.

   B. Preventive health care modalities must be inexpensive,
       convenient and accessible.

   C. There must be pervasive and persistent reinforcement of
       PHC activities. Motivation to continue participation
       must be maintained.

   D. Initial introduction of specific PHC modes or societal
       intervention should be developed in incremental steps or
       stages, for example, if mass disease specific screening
       in shopping malls is the objective, one disease should
       initially be introduced with others added individually or
       in logical clusters.

   E. Approaches must be segmental or stratified to meet the
       needs of high risk groups, to reach, initially, the most
       accessible segments and eventually, to pursue the harder
       to reach segments.

   F. Legal and licensing issues must be confronted in terms
       of medical practice laws governing specific modalities
       and innovations.

   G. Marketing strategies must take into consideration pre-
       vailing social conventions and mores. The scope of PHC
       may well include the promotion of self-examination for
       breast cancer or birth control information. Current
       problems with sex education in the schools should sensi-
       tize marketing to existent cross pressures. A related
       issue of the potential abuse and exploitation of relaxed

social mores was briefly mentioned.

In summary, a degree of optimism existed in the discussion in terms of the feasibility of marketing PHC, but it was felt that considerably more definition and specification of the possible modalities and levels of intervention were needed.

SUMMARY COMMENTS: PERCEPTIONS OF PROBLEMS AND LIMITATIONS OF PREVENTIVE HEALTH CARE AND MARKETING

Ronald G. Blankenbaker

Dr. Dale Achabal started discussion with a description of the problems and limitations encountered in the marketing of Health Maintenance organizations as an example of the difficulties anticipated with the marketing of preventive health care (See his text). This created a significant amount of discussion around the fact that the marketing of HMO's was involved primarily with the selling of memberships and that preventive medicine and quality of care was really a byproduct or indirect result. Consequently, the analogy is not necessarily a realistic one and the HMO model may not be useful for our purposes other than to try to learn from their mistakes. A further comment was that the purpose of HMO's was and is to provide earlier medical care and cost containment. Theoretically, this should coincide with appropriate preventive health care, but that is not an automatic assumption. A further comment was that the HMO is only one means of providing preventive health care and that we should be concerned with all means of providing such care and the marketing thereof.

Marketing of the HMO was described as being doomed to failure due to a lack of understanding and analysis of the consumer. The HMO concept was a mandate from the Federal government; the marketing of it was done without understanding of what was being sold and why, i.e., HMO's were sold and not marketed.

This brought up a more general discussion of some of the participants' concepts of marketing prior to the workshop being one of the 5th Avenue advertising firm stereotype which was not acceptable for use by the health profession. The workshop was successful in changing this stereotype to a better understanding of marketing as being a profession in itself which not only deals with advertising but more importantly with careful consumer analysis as to desires and needs along with the psychology by which a product can be made best available and useable by the consumer. This concept was felt quite acceptable to the health profession and indeed one which would be desirable to aid in the overall education of the public and improvement of health care.

Mr. Novelli then presented a quite interesting and provocative approach to the problems of marketing preventive health care. Of note here, he cautions us to remember that preventive health care is a mandate made by a Congress which tends to have a short attention span, that the evaluation of preventive health care marketing is quite difficult to measure, that preventive health care implies a changing of life styles which frequently has little consumer interest, that health care providers have a poor understanding of marketing and its techniques, that there are no standardized approaches and norms to "health marketing" and that the product (better health care) cannot be "shaped" or changed within our present means to become more palatable to the public.

Discussion then centered around the fact that health consumer research and analysis has no prior principles or standards to follow and we really don't know what questions to ask the consumer relative to his health. This brought up the thought that the atmosphere in which we work, i.e., the health care delivery system, may be too complex and therefore not conducive to marketing.

We then discussed whether or not a professional approach to marketing of preventive health care was a worthwhile endeavor, the consensus being that indeed it was. It was seen that once one has resolved the stigma of marketing as salesmanship only, that it then becomes an ally to the health professional and a welcome one at that.

As a personal sidelight, speaking as a practicing physician with a sincere interest in preventive medicine, this summarizer challenges the participants of the workshop and other interested individuals to develop procedures, standards, principles and additional models from which we can evaluate the capability of marketing principles to improve the overall health of this country via good preventive medicine. My personal bias is that we have to use every means at hand to "coerce" the public into good health practices, as general and even individual educational approaches to date have only met with somewhat limited success.

SUMMARY COMMENTS: PERCEPTIONS OF PROBLEMS AND LIMITATIONS OF PREVENTIVE HEALTH CARE AND MARKETING

Lawrence H. Wortzel

The group had an animated, far-ranging discussion during which many issues were raised, debated, contested, or digested. This summary attempts to list the issues that were covered and to present the essence of the discussion relating to each issue. The issues raised focused primarily on two broad topics: (1) the capacity of the present medical care payment and delivery system to foster preventive medical behavior, and (2) possible vehicles for accomplishing such behavior. Individual topics will be discussed more or less in the order listed above. Each could well be viewed as an interesting hypothesis, worthy of formal test.

I.   Present and emerging trends in payment for medical service do not foster preventive behavior on the part of payees.

The trends toward third party payment, and toward fixed cost schemes (Blue Cross-Blue Shield, HMOS) are viewed by consumers primarily as insurance against the cost of a serious medical problem. These schemes are not viewed primarily as opportunities for free or very low cost examinations for early disease detection, or even for free or low cost immunizations. These schemes are certainly not perceived by consumers as incentives to undertake preventive behavior or even to learn about such behavior.

First-dollar coverage, for example, removes all financial barriers to preventive services such as immunizations, but the demand for such services seems to be a function more of variables such as education and social class than of the presence of first-dollar coverage.

II.   The provider system is not set up to teach and encourage the practice of preventive medicine; it's set up to treat sick people. Fee-for-service organizations, of course, have traditionally been concerned primarily with treating the sick. But the HMO has been looked to as an organization to facilitate preventive care because it has, in theory, a steady, long-term constituency and some financial motivation. That is to say, an HMO that encourages preventive behavior among its patient group should eventually experience lower medical treatment costs.

In practice, however, the HMO may not really be encouraging such behavior. Any organization, whether profit-making or not-for-profit eventually seems to adopt a similar set of goals revolving about the ratios of its income to its expenses. HMOs appear to adopt short-term perspectives about the ratio of income to expense. To the extent an HMO does so, it is not likely to really encourage its patient population to come in for screenings or check-ups, let alone preventive health teaching. This is so because such activity raises costs in the short run, and any benefits that may accrue from such efforts only appear in the longer run. Perhaps what's needed is a change in the accounting system.

III. Existing health care providing organizations don't promote preventive care because the people in such organizations simply aren't oriented that way.

Physicians especially are oriented by medical school toward the treatment of acute conditions. When these physicians go out to practice, they are already socialized to the acute care "healer" role. In order to change the orientation of health care provider organizations, the orientation of the nation's medical schools must be changed to a preventive medicine orientation. Some schools in the allied health profession and in dentistry seem to be adopting this orientation, and it seems to change the procedures for dealing with patients.

IV. While delivery systems don't encourage preventive behavior, laws do encourage such behavior.

The major reason, for example, why children are immunized against certain diseases is primarily because the law requires such immunizations, rather than because parents want to protect their children.

V. The payoff in encouraging people to take preventive measures lies in manipulating (raising the salience of) non-health reasons for people to adopt such behavior.

Denying people access to services, applying social or psychological sanctions should encourage behavior such as non-smoking or getting immunized.

VI. There are vested interests that make it difficult to accomplish or even promote some preventive health behaviors.

The tobacco companies can still counter anti-smoking efforts with advertising and would make it virtually impossible to ban cigarettes from the market. Business interests make pollution control, even control of carcinogens quite difficult.

VIII. Workable systems may have to circumvent both the

physicians, and the environment.

On the other hand, we say "don't smoke." But, virtually wherever we go, there are ashtrays. We say "exercise more," but there are elevators, escalators and handy parking lots everywhere. We say "don't overeat" but high-calorie "junk" snack food confront us wherever we go.

VIII. One answer may be in "resocializing" people, or at least changing social norms.

The place to develop exercise norms may be in the schools. Perhaps every student should run two laps before class. The sports emphasis might be changed from team sports to life time participation sports. Teenage norms might be changed from "it's grown-up to smoke" to "it's grown-up not to smoke." More and more readily available exercising facilities might be provided.

IX. There are also potential political and economic solutions to preventive health problems.

When President Ford announced his swine flu program, it worked in reverse. The program was seen by many as politically motivated. Given a different political environment, such a program might have been received very positively.

We're experimenting with using economic incentives and disincentives to shape automobile purchase behavior. It's been used in India to encourage sterilization. To what extent can you use such incentives to encourage certain health related behaviors?

X. Consumer research has not reached the point of respectability at which it can be an indicator or determinant that will be used in designing programs, at least within the government.

Marketing researchers and some politicians (sometimes) will accept the results of a poll as a guideline to action but OMB, for example, will not. Too much of the government is unused to dealing with samples, and with attitudinal data.

XI. What are we marketing anyway? What's the product?

What the industry often markets isn't services, but is financial protection. When buying health insurance, people focus on protection rather than what they're entitled to. Insurance companies, especially, market protection rather than services.

Individual physicians, however, who operate on a fee-for-service basis, market their services through personal selling. But, it's still services rather than protection or prevention.

118

V.

IDENTIFYING CRITICAL ISSUES, OPPORTUNITIES AND
FUTURE RESEARCH AREAS FOR
MARKETING OF PREVENTIVE HEALTH CARE

This segment of the workshop was designed as a capstone. Its purpose was to bring together all of the parts that had been discussed in an attempt to assess the present position and chart future directions. Papers by Charles O. Crawford, Stanley G. House and William J. Kehoe comprise this segment of the Proceedings.

A REVIEW OF CRITICAL ISSUES AND OPPORTUNITIES
TO FURTHER THE DEVELOPMENT OF MARKETING AND
PREVENTIVE HEALTH CARE

Charles O. Crawford

OVERVIEW OF THE CONFERENCE AND PROBLEMS IDENTIFIED

There was a great deal of testimony to the fact that the conference was very stimulating, very enlightening and created an aura of euphoria. This feeling of enlightenment and stimulation was expressed by a number of persons at various points in this final session. However, the group euphoria sometimes can dissipate quickly when participants return to their regular jobs and the pressures of those regular jobs. Along these same lines it was emphasized that the session regarding the perceptions of problems and limitations of Marketing Preventive Health Care provided a real opportunity for good solid discussion on a multi-disciplinary approach to the problem of marketing or getting people to adopt preventive health behaviors. A point which was raised a number of times was that there is a need to take a hard look at where such marketing and/or health education efforts should take place. Should it be in the schools, at shopping malls, with varying kinds of audiences, and/or with other considerations in mind? It seems that there was a very clear recognition of the importance of market segmentation or the need for clear delineation of target audiences for health education programming. Consideration needs to be given to whether marketing theory and techniques can actually lend themselves to the marketing of services where concepts and knowledge change are the important components rather than some commercial good around which marketing theory and technique have been built in the past.

Several points summarizing the problems were made. For example, the mass advertising success of health marketing may

119

perhaps have been unsuccessful because the emphasis was on a product and not on a brand of that product, to use marketing terminology. The structure appears to be irrelevant to bringing about changes in preventive health behavior; what is important are the educational and socio-economic factors. What really has been sold up to now is financial protection or insurance, not services. In fact some persons pay their premium in anticipation of having their financial problems taken care of without knowing the bundle of services for which they were paying.

One point which had been made at a number of points throughout the day and a half conference was that a variety of incentives are needed to get people to engage in or adopt preventive health care behaviors. These are: (1) environmental incentives such as removing ashtrays in rooms to reduce the chances of smoking, (2) altering peer influence in smoking so that the emphasis is on nonsmoking as the thing to do, rather than as smoking as the thing to do, (3) various types of economic incentives to get people to adopt preventive health behaviors, (4) impose government regulations such as those outlined in Dr. Hochbaum's paper, i.e., forms of passive health action like the air bags on cars, and (5) limitations to institutional access such as requiring certain immunizations before a young child can be admitted to schools. The point was also made that it was important that efforts should be made to get medical schools to emphasize prevention more in their education programs. Additional aspects of importance include keeping constantly in mind that it is not necessary and very often not feasible to shoot for 100% adoption of any given health behavior. Another aspect to be considered is the acknowledgement of the hospital as a provider of preventive health behavior. It could be utilized as a very positive force in bringing about preventive health care.

A perhaps obvious but underemphasized key in this behavior change is the physician. While their medical training does not focus on preventive health behavior, they must be involved in planning any changes in strategy. This serves two objectives. First, by involving them, their sensitivities may be increased toward the importance of preventive behavior. Secondly, if they are involved in planning, then the commitment to follow through might be strengthened.

WHAT ARE THE OPPORTUNITIES FOR FUTURE ACTION

The question now is where do we go from here and what further actions need to be taken? A follow-up should be involved with struggling with specific concrete problems including the analysis of these problems and proposed solutions. A potential for leadership in identifying and supporting work in this area is the relatively new Bureau of Health Education of the CDC in Atlanta. Another possibility is the emerging Office of Health Information and Health Promotion, in D.C. A possibility for a specific program might be to develop what could be called educational packages which could be made available to school health personnel and physicians to work singly or in groups with individuals charged with a marketing or health education function. In doing this we need to keep in mind the geographical differences in the personnel who would be involved in the delivery process. In short, what is being described is the process of market segmentation.

An observation made and an opinion expressed by one participant was that what had happened in the workshop was that it was a behavioral change process as much as being about behavioral change processes, and that it was unfortunate that government agencies were not present which have a bearing in the environmental context in which individuals must make decisions about such matters related to preventive health care behavior. Agencies might have included the F.D.A., F.T.C., and others. The point was made that the workshop was deliberately kept small to facilitate discussion. The opportunity for future sessions is present and should include not only those agencies but possibly congressmen and congresswomen.

The potential for the compilation and development down the road of a series of case studies which would demonstrate how marketing has been involved in bringing about changes in preventive health behavior is an obvious opportunity that had not been done to the best of knowledge of several participants. Several mentioned that they searched for such a compilation of case studies but could not find any in the literature.

People in marketing are very good at looking at the conditions under which advertising and personal selling are effective. What is needed now is to settle down and work out some kind of a system for preventive health behavior change. One of the underlying questions of the workshop was--what works? Everything seems to work a little, even doing nothing. What needs to be done is to systematically "pile up" these many and varied bits of information which we have. All of the workshop participants and many others are doing something back at their respective home stations and what is needed is to continue to do this, evaluate what is being done, and report it so that it can be systematically compiled. One way of doing this is the development of case studies.

At this point in the emerging union between marketing and preventive health care, the development of a project would be helpful to carry the impetus of this initial step. An interdisciplinary task force might pull together all the information presented at the workshop and develop such a project. However, the question remains--what is it that is going to be subjected to marketing processes. We need to be very specific if we are going to develop a project. For example, concentration on nutrition change might be appropriate. However, choosing to focus on "mechanisms" for carrying out the marketing or educational campaign can be dangerous. Marketing, in one sense, is offering people a chance to decide what they prefer to die from. If the person wants to take all of the steps to reduce the risk of heart disease, and is successful in this, then that person might well die of cancer. If he or she takes all the steps to reduce the risks from both of these diseases, and is successful, then perhaps the cause of death might be diabetes or some other chronic and insidious disease. There appears to be a "following of the band wagon" in this country with regard to the whole emphasis on self care. Consequently, what is needed is a specific or a bullet approach rather than using a shotgun approach to cover the waterfront. In other words, concern should be switched from the product to the brand or the specific health behavior to be changed.

CONCLUSION

To summarize, it is quite apparent that not only did those participating in the workshop gain a great deal from the interdisciplinary approach and the emphasis on the potential role that marketing can play in preventive health care, but there now is an obvious need to sensitize others in the medical profession, the marketing profession, the health education profession, etc. to the issues raised in this workshop. The point was made that health people need to learn more from marketing people and marketing people need to learn more from the health people.

The question remains as to the effective ways to bring this about. One possible way to accomplish the objective plus facilitate communication and interchange of experiences among the present workshop participants would be to develop a newsletter. Another more popular possibility would be the development of additional conferences. If this was to be done, it would help to develop a clear focus if a specific topic (like immunization) were chosen for emphasis. The Bureau of Health Education would be a potential source for help to organize the structure and procedure for such an interchange.

THE FUTURE WILL BE GUIDED BY BETTER DEFINITIONS

Stanley G. House

It was clear that the stated comments and conclusions of were in harmony of the main tenor of the several preceding open sessions and private conversations throughout the Conference as summarized in Dr. Crawfords review.,

Additional points to be made include a greater emphasis on more functional definitions of "Preventive Health Care". The term is not yet alike perceived by doctors, health professionals, educators, government bureaucrats, politicians, editorialists, sick patients or well consumers. Its meaning depends on who is using it, to whom it is being addressed, and for the purpose intended; but thus far, the term itself is struggling to surmount a variety of perspectives.

On the other hand, "marketing" is quite well defined -- with its procedures of program design, testing and application systematically organized and widely recognized. Questions as to novel economic theory and as to the validity of assumptions do not question the basic principles of marketing; rather, they reflect debate as to the tools of particular marketing efforts.

From a traditionalist point of view, applying marketing principles to "Preventive Health Care" should only be another classic exercise of "Have problem, can solve." However, what is the problem? Does "Preventive Health" care exclude non-medical methods, such as life-style modification? Does it include societal imperatives? Is "Preventive Health Care" either quantitatively or qualitatively measurable, except in manpower/hours/dollars terms? What are the "norms" of this subject? The answers to these kinds of questions should be settled, by and large, in order for marketing to get a respectable handle on Preventive Health Care."

As a beginning toward a marketing understanding of "Preventive Health Care," the following initiatory steps could be considered by all interested parties:

a. Each of us should accept a personal role as part of an informed health "team" in our family.

b. Each of us should advocate and practice education-medicine (health activation) in our community.

c. Each of us should monitor health care provider

123

systems, analyze the on-going results and report thereon.

d. Each of us should keep searching for organizations (private and public) that seek to involve the population in political/social awareness of health problems and lend our support thereto.

The above experiences, collectively and continually gathered and evaluated, would probably lead to the meaningful working definitions of "Preventive Health Care" necessary for marketing purposes.

CONCEPTUALIZING THE INTEGRATION OF MARKETING
AND PREVENTIVE HEALTH CARE

William J. Kehoe

SESSION OVERVIEW

The participants unanimously extolled the meaningfulness of the workshop and the dialogue that had been opened across disciplinary lines. The importance of that dialogue was noted by many of the participants and the health educators, particularly, expressed the opinion that the workshop had reconceptualized their understanding of the concept of marketing and its potential contribution to preventive health care. The expression was that, as a group, the participants were beyond conceptualizing marketing as promotion or selling and had recognized that marketing was a means to affect behavioral change. As such, it has a potential and a significant contribution to make in the health area. Those in marketing are generally good empiricists, skilled at problem conceptualization, and with significant operational skills in assessing an environment, understanding its behavioral underpinnings and applying appropriate marketing technology to affect change. As the health educator is concerned with affecting change, the linkage of marketing and preventive health care is conceptually axiomatic.

HISTORICAL HEALTH CARE ANTECEDENTS TO MARKETING'S ENTRY

In a historical sense, it was noted that the health care area has experienced significant changes in its corporate mission during this century. From the early part of the century to the late 1950's, the mission was one of a curative nature. The emphasis was on curing disease in the presence of symptomatic indicators of a disease. During the 1960's, the mission evolved to a "take care of everyone" posture in a preventive mode. The treatment focus changed symptomatic treatment of disease to asymptomatic care. It was not until the 1970's that the cost benefits of preventive care were given serious consideration. Preventive medicine is a way of controlling cost. Marketing, through its persuasive information dimension, can make decided cost contributions by effectively providing the means for the health provider and the consumer to communicate, to know and to interact with each other, thereby ensuring for behavioral change on the part of the consumer to a preventive health care regimen. And, once the regimen is established, marketing technology is useful to reinforce the preventive decision and to reduce any cognitive dissonance that may ensue.

125

There was a generally expressed need for a sharing of the workshop experience with others in the health education and marketing disciplines, as well as for continuing the integrative thrust established in the workshop. Discussion of methods to share the experience and continue the thrust ensued at both the macro and more micro levels.

Macro Discussion

At this level, discussion centered on the broader methods of maintaining the spirit of the workshop. Prescriptions ranged from the very pragmatic "do it" to more thoroughly discussed and conceptualized proposals.

Joining each other's associations was suggested as a means of sharing the workshop experience and enlarging individual spheres of contact. Coupled with this was discussion of the workshop entity affiliating with an already established professional association in order to establish a base and address the content of the workshop to wider audiences. Caveats to this proposal centered around the fact that the workshop group might become lost or engulfed by established associations.

Publication of the Proceedings was recognized as the primarly vehicle of sharing the workshop experience. In addition, most participants expressed the desire for additional workshops in the area and endorsed the proposal of the formation of a task force charged with the responsibility of establishing methods to share the experience of the workshop. It was suggested that the task force be tentatively titled the "Select Task Force On Applying Marketing In The Preventive Health Area".

Micro Discussion

In addition to discussion of professional affiliation, establishing a task force and publishing the Proceedings, more micro and specific suggestions were made for the future. These involved the development of educational packages and case studies among others.

The group noted that several new federal agencies had been established that might be utilized to ensure for the continuing dialogue and integration between health care and marketing. These included the Bureau of Health Education at the Center for Disease Control in Atlanta and the Office Of Health Information And Health Promotion in Washington, D.C.

Marketing segmentation as a tool for continuing the inte-

126

gration was also discussed. The suggestion was made that education packages be developed, recognizing differences in audiences, geography, and etc., and made available to physicians, health maintenance organization personnel, and school health officials charged with the health education of behavioral change function. While appealing from a contribution of marketing to health care viewpoint, this was recognized as an operational tool (which is needed in the health communications area) but not as a specific vehicle for expanding the product of the workshop.

Case studies were also suggested in which operational examples of marketing's involvement in behavioral health change would be demonstrated. This idea was recognized of merit, but necessarily difficult to complete in the short run. Rather, it is an excellent long run mechanism for communicating examples of effective integration of marketing and health care.

Also noted was the necessity of compiling the many bits of information all the workshop participants possessed on what was currently being done in the marketing/health care area, together with feedback on the effectiveness of these activities. This is a descriptive prescription, and description is an appropriate first step in any emerging area. While an appropriate suggestion, an operational mechanism or clearinghouse for the information was not specific by the group. Perhaps, the task force or the editors of these Proceedings are appropriate clearing house mechanisms.

CONCLUSION

As the session ended, there was a resolve to maintain the unique product of the workshop. An interdisciplinary dialogue had been opened and an awareness of the mutuality and potential contributions to be made between preventive health care and marketing was more fully understood. A commitment to sensitize others in marketing, health education and medicine to the emerging integration of marketing and health care was shared by all participants. This Summarizer sensed a group feeling of being at the start of an emerging, dynamic and exciting new era for marketing and preventive health care.

VI

REFLECTIONS

To conclude the Proceedings, a paper, jointly authored by the three workshop co-chairpersons, is presented. It addresses their reflections on marketing preventive health care.

REFLECTIONS ON MARKETING PREVENTIVE HEALTH CARE

Patrick E. Murphy, Philip D. Cooper and William J. Kehoe

The diversity of papers contained in this proceedings and the infancy of this area make it impossible to definitively discuss the absolute status of marketing preventive health care. Therefore, the major purpose of this section is to synthesize the progress on the subject. Initially, marketing's application to the health care industry is examined. Then, the notion of market segmentation and its relationship to health services consumers is discussed. The marketing mix elements (e.g., product, price, promotion and channels of distribution) which interface with preventive health care are presented. Finally, the external environments (i.e., forces) affecting preventive health care marketing are briefly summarized.

MARKETING'S APPLICATION

Voluntary exchange relationships between two parties represent the focal point of marketing. Since providers of preventive health care services and consumers of these services expect to benefit from the exchange, it appears that this relationship comes under the purview of marketing. Specifically, the providers hope to gain financial and psychic rewards from keeping the consumer healthy and the buyer in turn anticipates comprehensive health services when needed at a lower cost. Although Dr. Hochbaum (see "A Critical Assessment of Marketing's Place in Preventive Health Care" in this volume) perceptively noted several differences between the marketing of economic goods and services and health care, the primary requirement of marketing (i.e., exchange) seems to be met in the health services sector.

MARKET SEGMENTATION AND CONSUMER BEHAVIOR

Just as no commercial product appeals to all 216 million U.S. consumers, the market for preventive health care services is also "segmented". Many segmentation possibilities exist for preventive health care marketers. Consumers' location, family

128

status and life cycle stage, etc. are useful bases for segmenting the market. For instance, Dr. Cooper (see "A Consumer Perspective on Preventive Service Usage" in this volume) reported that attitudes toward service usage and normative influences may provide potentially useful segmentation guidelines. The important criterion that marketers of preventive health care need to keep in mind is that a successful overall marketing strategy begins with proper market segmentation.

The internal and external variables affecting consumer decision making warrant study of health care management. Basic principles of motivation, perception, learning, personality, attitudes and attitude change (i.e., internal variables) offer insights into all consumption behavior including health. One internal variable, expectations, has not received much attention in the consumer behavior literature, but may be particularly useful in explaining health behavior. Because of nearly universal insurance coverage and advances in medical technology, health care consumers may be considered to possibly "expect" the most expensive and thorough treatment. Preventive health care marketers must try to alter these expectations by showing that these costly procedures are no substitute for a healthy lifestyle. In addition, the external variables of culture, social class, reference group membership, and family background influence an individual's health-related behavior.

MARKETING MIX VARIABLES

The first variable to be discussed is product. In the case of health care, the product is conceptualized as a bundle of services. The difference between the consumer and marketer's view of product is important to recognize. Consumers are buying "benefits" derived from health services such as vigor, beauty and a long active life. The providers of preventive health care are offering a range of specialties including all inpatient and outpatient care. A provider with a marketing point of view would focus on providing the bundle of services which help the consumers achieve the benefits they are seeking.

The pricing practices of preventive health care marketers do not usually follow classic marketing principles. Prices in the traditional fee-for-service system are often set for a specified period at a particular amount with the only difference being between an individual and family plans. Policies such as price lining for different levels of service (i.e., comprehensive, limited or catastrophic care) and price adjustments for those who utilize services infrequently need to be studied. Also, more data about the prices of the specific services is necessary for consumers to make informed choices. While the concept of prepaid group practice has been espoused for some time, this form of delivery has not been widely accepted compared to the traditional fee for service system. If this does find wider acceptance, it will have a dramatic effect on pricing as well as an influence on encouraging a higher level of preventive health care.

The technique used for informing as well as persuading and reminding buyers is called <u>promotion</u>. Promotion, which includes primarily personal selling and advertising, is marketing's most visible activity. Even more basic than informing consumers about prices is educating them concerning the concept of preventive care. Since the health care system has traditionally been oriented toward acute, crisis-oriented care, substantial promotional activity will be necessary. Advertising compaigns are currently being used by some hospitals and HMO's, but little intensive mass media advertising has been undertaken to date. An example of a specific communication strategy for family planning is provided by Dr. Kar (see "Communications and Marketing in Health and Family Planning Programs" in this volume).

Personal selling efforts for preventive care have largely been left to the insurance companies such as the Blues, whose salespersons are charged with promoting the program. However, physicians associated with HMO's or Free Medical Clinics seem to be uniquely suited to undertaking a part-time personal selling role. Since they are the most knowledgeable sources available, their efforts, either one-to-one with a patient or before groups, would probably be quite effective. Thus, promoting preventive health care will provide a major challenge to all individuals involved.

The channel of <u>distribution</u> is concerned with the actual delivery of the health services. Many institutions such as hospitals, clinics and physicians' offices are associated with the system. If preventive care is to have a pervasive effect on the population, new avenues for delivery will need experimentation. Professor Venkatesan provides several innovative suggestions in his presentation which is included in this volume. Because health care is a service, the channel is a direct one between producer and consumer. It is not possible to warehouse services, therefore, efficient utilization of human and technical resources is imperative.

From the above discussion it is hopefully evident that the marketing mix variables can be applied to preventive health care. To develop a successful program all of the mix elements must be coordinated. The strategic implication for marketers of these services is to understand the dynamics of these variables and how they relate to satisfy customer satisfaction.

Since marketing activities do not take place in a vacuum, several external environments are relevant to this analysis. Although Dr. Chamberlain presented an overview of the environment in this volume, a brief discussion is also included here. Specifically, the environmental aspects which warrant further consideration are the government, technology, competition and ethics.

Government, at all levels, is becoming a more pervasive force affecting the marketing of products and services. Combined with the regulations concerning the health care area, marketers of preventive health services have a formidable task in responding to governmental influences. Some of the current governmental problems were analyzed by Flexner, Schoeni and Ward in their position papers. The possibility of a national health insurance program may have a significant impact on preventive health care. Hence, marketers must be adaptable to the restrictions or incentives placed on them by government.

Technology and competition are additional environmental forces that preventive health care marketers must take into account. Technological developments in medical equipment field have greatly increased the sophistication of the study of medicine. Preventive care practitioners, therefore, need to keep abreast of the latest technological breakthroughs. However, caution should be exercised in the dependence on technology to solve problems rather than common sense approaches to lifestyle. Also, competition by the traditional elements of the health care delivery system will provide formidable opposition to preventive plans. Managers of these plans must study their competition to capitalize on the unique advantages that they offer consumers. Just as the governmental environment is a changing one, the areas of technology and competition are also dynamic.

Finally, the ethical environment facing preventive health care marketers deserves attention. Although the subject was broached, in reference to advertising, and is reviewed by Dr. Moriarity in this volume, the fact that ethics pervade all marketing activities must be recognized. It is essential that preventive health care marketers avoid the ethical pitfalls that have plagued commercial product marketers. If marketing is to play a positive role in furthering the cause of preventive medicine, the ethical dimensions of all related marketing activities must be satisfied.

CONCLUSION

Although these reflections have taken a cursory view of

marketing preventive health care, the framework presented encompassed the relevant issues. It can be concluded that marketing is a pervasive activity focusing on exchange relationships and it is an appropriate tool to be used by preventive health care practitioners.

The fact that the consumer should be the focal point of all marketing strategy is hopefully evident. Since all consumers cannot be realistically satisfied by preventive health marketers, the psychological, sociological and behavioral attributes of the most promising segments should be analyzed. Interactions among the marketing mix elements -- product, price promotion and channels -- needs coordination and the overall objective should be to create a synergistic effect. The governmental, technological, competitive and ethical environments also place constraints on the marketer of preventive health care services.

In conclusion, the task facing those marketing preventive health care is a formidable, but not an unachievable, one.